THE COMPREHENSIVE GUIDE TO SKIN CARE

THE COMPREHENSIVE GUIDE TO SKIN CARE

FROM ACNE TO WRINKLES, WHAT TO DO (AND NOT DO) TO STAY HEALTHY AND LOOK YOUR BEST

REBECCA B. CAMPEN, M.D.

PRAEGER
An Imprint of ABC-CLIO, LLC

A B C ☰ C L I O

Santa Barbara, California • Denver, Colorado • Oxford, England

Library of Congress Cataloging-in-Publication Data

Campen, Rebecca B.
  The comprehensive guide to skin care : from acne to wrinkles, what to do (and not do)
  to stay healthy and look your best / Rebecca B. Campen.
    p. cm.
  Includes bibliographical references and index.
    ISBN 978–0–313–37886–7 (hard copy : alk. paper) — ISBN 978–0–313–37887–4
(ebook)
1. Skin—Care and hygiene. 2. Self-care, Health. 3. Beauty, Personal. I. Title.
RL87.C365   2010
646.7′26—dc22   2009034153

14 13 12 11 10   1 2 3 4 5

This book is also available on the World Wide Web as an eBook.
Visit www.abc-clio.com for details.

ABC-CLIO, LLC
130 Cremona Drive, P.O. Box 1911
Santa Barbara, California 93116-1911

This book is printed on acid-free paper (∞)

Manufactured in the United States of America

CONTENTS

PART I: THE TRUTH   1
  1. Getting on the Right Track   3
  2. Successful People Have Good Skin   7
  3. Getting Started: You, Too, Can Have Beautiful Skin   9
  4. Special Care for Hands, Feet, Nails, Hair, Lips, and Elbows   17
  5. Seven Secrets for Sensational Skin   23
  6. Your Amazing Skin   27
  7. When Skin Ages: The Scientific Basis   35
  8. Amazing Transformations in Your Appearance   39
  9. Protect Your Child's Skin   53

PART II: SORTING TRUTH FROM HYPE   55
  10. Advertisements or Truths?   57
  11. Getting Past the Myths and Hang-Ups   63
  12. Alternative Therapies, Natural Products, Fact or Fiction?   67
  13. New "Breakthrough Products": Do They Work?   73

PART III: A SKIN CARE PROGRAM FOR YOUR SKIN   77
  14. The Healthy Skin Program   79

PART IV: SKIN PROBLEMS   97
  15. What You Need to Know About Skin Cancer   99
  16. Dry Skin, Chapped Lips, and Mottled Skin   109
  17. Problems with Hair and Scalp   111
  18. Acne, Rosacea, and Other Facial Blemishes   117
  19. Those Awful Warts!   127
  20. Bites and Infestations   131
  21. Unwanted Spots and Growths   135
  22. Rash   139
  23. Skin Infections   145
  24. Other Annoying Problems   151
  25. Chronic Skin Problems   157

26. Problems In and Around the Mouth   161
27. Skin Changes in Pregnancy   163
28. Common Problems in Children   165

PART V: THE FUTURE   169
29. Oh Crystal Ball, What Is the Future for Us All?   171
30. Hot Areas of Scientific Research That Will Change Skin Care   175
31. New Breakthroughs   179
32. Learning from the Simplest Organisms   193
33. The New Genomic Era—How It Will Impact Skin Care   199
34. Renewing Our Body: Stem Cells and Tissue Transplantation   203
35. Tissue Engineering—Making a New Body Part   207
36. Nanotechnology—A Whole New World   209
37. Medical Tourism—A Vacation and a Face Lift?   213
38. Taking Technology Home   215
39. The Case for Vitamin D   217
40. The Finishing Touch   219

Appendix   221

Notes   229

References   241

Index   243

PART I

THE TRUTH

CHAPTER 1

GETTING ON THE
RIGHT TRACK

Tears streamed down Mary's cheeks as she sat on the exam table. I hardly recognized her. Her face was so blistered and swollen that her eyes were tiny slits. I handed her a tissue.

"Mary! What happened!"

Mary dabbed gingerly at the sides of her eyes with the tissue. Her voice shook.

"I'm supposed to be getting married next week . . ." she sobbed. *"The last three months has been so hectic. With all the planning, I haven't had time to get myself ready for the wedding except to pick out the wedding gown. I—I wanted to look my best . . . so two days ago I went for a beauty consultation at my favorite department store. The beauty consultant said that I should start my marriage off on the right foot with the best skin care . . . I bought everything that she recommended . . . exfoliant, astringent, toner, creams—everything! It all cost a fortune, but I thought I was doing the right thing . . . Today I woke up looking like this! Now everything is ruined! How can I walk down the aisle like this!"*

Fortunately, Mary's dilemma had a happy ending. With treatment her skin was radiant in time for her walk down the aisle. And she learned what her skin really needs to keep it youthful and healthy—and what it doesn't need!

What *is* the right thing to do for your skin? Should you use exfoliants, astringents, peels, toners, eye creams, night creams? Should you use antiwrinkle creams now to prevent wrinkles later or to treat wrinkles now? What about photofacials, microdermabrasion, and facial peels? Do they improve skin health and appearance? What is *really* necessary for good skin care?

I'm a dermatologist at Massachusetts General Hospital, a teaching hospital of Harvard Medical School. People come from all over the world to Massachusetts General Hospital for treatment of skin problems. Every skin problem is different. But everyone wants to know what is really true about good skin care.

Billions of dollars are spent each year by consumers relying on skin care products advertised to perform miracles that don't happen, while inexpensive products found in drug stores often work just as well as highly promoted, expensive products. This book is for you to know what is really true about skin care and what your skin really needs.

You will learn:

- What your skin needs and doesn't need
- What *to* do about wrinkles
- How to get rid of dark spots
- How sun really affects skin
- What to do about adult acne
- Which skin changes may signal skin cancer
- What to do about large pores
- How to reduce facial redness
- What types of sunscreens are best
- How to *prevent* wrinkles
- What really works to make skin look younger
- And many other topics important to skin care and appearance

This book will help you determine the particular needs for your skin type and set goals for your appearance. It will help you design a plan to make your skin look and feel beautiful and healthy.

The book is divided into five parts. Part I (Chapters 1 through 9) introduces you to good skin care and discusses cosmetic procedures that can erase years from your skin. Part II (Chapters 10 through 13) shows you how to tell truth from advertising hype. Part III (Chapter 14) helps you determine your skin type to develop a skin care program tailored to your skin. Part IV (Chapters 15 through 28) discusses common skin problems. Part V (Chapters 29 through 40) reveals what's new in skin care now and what's coming in the near future based on scientific discoveries today.

- In Chapter 2, you'll learn the basics for good skin care.
- In Chapter 3, you'll learn the Golden Rule for beautiful skin.
- In Chapter 4, you'll learn how to give special care for hands, feet, nails, hair, lips, and elbows.
- In Chapter 5, you'll learn Seven Secrets for Sensational Skin.
- In Chapter 6, you'll learn what goes on inside skin.
- In Chapter 7, you'll learn what happens when skin ages.
- In Chapter 8, you'll learn what you can do *now* about skin aging.
- In Chapter 9, you'll learn how to protect your baby's skin.
- Chapter 10 will reveal how to sort truth from hype.
- Chapter 11 will dispel myths about skin care.
- In Chapter 12, you'll learn what's true and what's not true about herbs, vitamins, and "Natural" products.
- In Chapter 13, you'll learn about new "breakthrough" products and whether they really work.

- In Chapter 14, you'll be introduced to the Healthy Skin Care Program, a program designed for your own skin type and skin problems.
- In Chapter 15, you'll learn signs of skin cancer.
- In Chapter 16, you'll learn what to do about dry skin, chapped lips, and mottled skin.
- In Chapter 17, you'll learn how to handle problems with hair and scalp.
- In Chapter 18, you'll learn what to do about acne, rosacea, and other facial blemishes.
- Chapter 19 will tell you how to treat warts.
- In Chapter 20, you'll learn what to do about spider and mite bites.
- Chapter 21 will discuss treatment of unwanted spots and growths that come with aging.
- In Chapter 22, you'll learn about skin rashes.
- In Chapter 23, you'll learn about skin infections and treatments.
- In Chapter 24, you'll learn what to do about annoying problems such as itching or excessive sweating.
- In Chapter 25, you'll learn about treatment of chronic problems such as psoriasis.
- Chapter 26 will discuss cold sores, canker sores, and other problems in and around the mouth.
- Chapter 27 will discuss skin changes during pregnancy.
- Chapter 28 will discuss common problems in children.
- Chapter 29 will discuss what's in the future for skin care based on scientific discoveries today.
- Chapter 30 will reveal hot areas of scientific research that will change skin care.
- Chapter 31 will discuss new breakthroughs today in skin care.
- Chapter 32 will discuss what we are learning from the simplest organisms that will impact skin care in the future
- Chapter 33 will reveal what the New Genomic Era will bring to skin care.
- In Chapter 34, you will learn about the cells that keep our skin renewed.
- In Chapter 35, you will learn how scientists are learning to make new body parts.
- In Chapter 36, you will be introduced to the amazing world of nanotechnology.
- In Chapter 37, you will learn about "medical tourism," a money-making endeavor in many countries.
- Chapter 38 discusses new at-home laser treatments for scalp and hair removal.
- Chapter 39 discusses the controversy between wearing sunscreen and getting enough Vitamin D.
- Chapter 40 discusses the finishing touch!

CHAPTER 2

SUCCESSFUL PEOPLE HAVE GOOD SKIN

Have you ever noticed that everyone on television—or in the movies—has beautiful skin? Of course there are ways to create that illusion on the screen. But in real life you've also noticed that men and women of power always have blemish-free skin.

Imagine yourself in a board room—a long table with 16 people around the table. Your eye goes to the people in the center or at the end—they are likely to be the people of power around the table. What do they look like in your imagination? Do they have a scarred face? Perhaps. What about a red, blemished face. Unlikely. Most often you will imagine a smooth-complexion and a blemish-free face. That is because the power figures that we see in real life usually have this appearance. They carry themselves with confidence. They know that they look good, they feel good, and they feel powerful.

A clear complexion and a healthy body give confidence. You know that you have been effective in making your appearance as pleasant and dynamic as possible, and you know that you will be just as effective in the boardroom as in any other setting.

IS YOUR SKIN AT ITS BEST?

Look in the mirror. Is your skin firm, glowing with health, blemish-free? Is your color healthy or sallow? Does your natural skin show its true beauty or is your skin smeared with foundation makeup? Is your forehead youthful, or do frown lines crease your brow? Is your skin smooth, or are there growths that you would just as soon do without?

WHY WORRY ABOUT SKIN?

Three reasons:

(1) We are vain. We like people to admire us, and they are more likely to do so if we have good skin.
(2) Good skin reflects a healthy body. A healthy body makes us happier and more effective.
(3) Good skin gives us confidence and helps us succeed. Successful people have good skin

This book will tell you what you need to know to make your skin as blemish-free and attractive as possible. The book will dispel myths and discuss the most recent techniques for changing appearance and creating the look that you want to have. You'll learn side effects as well as benefits of procedures so that your decisions can be based on the true story. You'll learn new scientific discoveries that are taking us into a revolutionary new realm of skin care.

CHAPTER 3

GETTING STARTED: YOU, TOO, CAN HAVE BEAUTIFUL SKIN

I'm so confused. Do I need a day lotion and a night cream? And do I need a separate cream for around my eyes. I hear that alpha-hydroxy acids are important. And what about my astringent and the clarifying lotion? Which do I put on first?

—Diane, age 23

The first thing to do is to take a deep breath, exhale slowly, and put aside all of your products. Yes—that's right. Put them all aside. Start with a clean slate.

First you're going to learn the Basics for Beautiful Skin. They are the foundation for your own skin care regimen. *The basics are all that you really need for daily care of normal skin.*[1] Anything else is extra.

What are the Basics?

The Basics are (1) a mild soap for cleansing your skin, (2) a moisturizer if your skin is dry, and (3) sun protection.

MILD SOAP

I'm very careful about my skin. I never put soap on my face. I just rinse with water. I use a cleansing cream to clean my face. So why am I getting all of these clogged pores?

—Rachael, age 28

Cleanse your face daily. Use a gentle, unscented soap[2] and rinse well. Water alone won't do. Do not rely on cleansing creams to clean your face. Creams can clog pores and cause problems. Makeup left on overnight also clogs pores and causes blemishes.

> **BASICS FOR BEAUTIFUL SKIN**
>
> (1) Mild soap for cleansing your skin
> (2) Moisturizer after cleansing your skin, if your skin is dry
> (3) Sun protection

I buy only the best soaps and moisturizers—I get my soap from the Natural Products store—it has soothing oil from the cannonberry tree and is very mild—and I order my moisturizer from Paris. I've never had any problems with my skin before so why now? Something else must be irritating my face.

—Linda, age 38

You can develop sensitivity to a product even though you have been using it for a long time without problems. One day you apply your favorite cream or moisturizer or makeup product that you have used forever, and to your horror, your face turns beet red! It can happen. If it does, don't rule out your favorite product just because you've always used it. If any product, expensive or not, causes irritation, stop using it immediately. If a product usually considered mild irritates your skin, avoid using it.[3]

The truth is that you don't need to buy special soap, moisturizers, and sunscreens. You can find what you need at the drugstore, supermarket, or discount store. We'll discuss this further in the next few pages.

I work in a hospital, so I like to use antibacterial soap to wash my face at night. I scrub it clean with a washcloth. But my face looks rough and red all the time.

—Miriam, age 45

If you prefer antibacterial soap, make sure that it doesn't irritate your skin, which can happen. Rough, red skin can be a portal to bacteria, and infection can occur. If your skin is sensitive, you are better off with a mild soap that doesn't irritate your skin and open it to infection. You can get mild soaps such as Dove for Sensitive Skin and Cetaphil Soap from the drugstore.

When you wash your face, do so gently, preferably with your hands. Don't scrub or use abrasive materials to routinely clean your face. Washcloths often harbor a residue of detergent that can irritate your skin. Rinse your face well, and pat dry with a terrycloth towel. Apply a moisturizer if your skin is dry. You can get good, unscented moisturizers, such as Moisturel Lotion or Lubriderm Lotion, from the drugstore.

But I have to use cleansing cream to get my makeup off. There's no way that soap will get it all off. And I can't leave off my makeup with all these acne bumps all over my face!

—Cheryl, age 40

Foundation makeup is the worst possible thing that you can apply to your face when you have acne. But it's natural to feel that you can't possibly leave the house without your makeup when your face is broken out with acne! It is very important to *clear your skin blemishes with the help of a dermatologist* and avoid wearing foundation whenever possible so that your skin can "breathe."

If you feel that you must wear foundation makeup until your face clears, be sure that it is has a *water-base* and is *oil-free*. You won't need cleansing creams to remove water-base foundation—a mild soap will do. Purpose Soap is effective in removing water-base makeup and also helps treat acne. Cleansing creams make acne worse. As your face clears, use spot cover-sticks or medicated acne cover-ups as necessary.

I have the most wonderful soap—it smells like orange blossoms. I have the bath oil, too, and I relish my "down time" in the tub after a long day at work. But lately I've been itching all over.

—Sandra, age 33

We all love perfumed soaps. But unfortunately perfume is the number-one irritant of skin. If you're using perfumed soaps and not having any skin problems, keep on enjoying that soap and the bath oil, too. But at the first sign of skin irritation—and that includes itching—stop using your perfumed soaps and bath oils. They are the likely culprits. Go Back To The Basics and use an unscented soap like Dove Soap or Cetaphil Soap.

MOISTURIZER

I spent a fortune on this moisturizer that is supposed to replenish moisture in my skin. I can't use most moisturizers because my skin is oily—but this one is especially for oily skin. And it smells so good. It's sold through my doctor's office.

—Amanda, age 50

Several things should set off the "hype" alarm for you here—even though this is sold through your doctor's office. *Moisturizers don't put water into skin. They maintain the moisture that's already in skin* by protecting the skin barrier. This keeps skin smooth and soft. Most moisturizers contain water, lipids, emulsifiers, and preservatives, but they may also contain fragrance and other additives such as vitamins, minerals, various "natural extracts," and sunscreens. A moisturizer should be *simple, without fragrance or many additives.* The more additives, the more possibilities for allergic or irritant reactions.

If you don't have dry skin, you don't need a moisturizer. You are more likely to need a moisturizer in the winter when indoor air is warm and dry or as you grow older and your skin loses some of its natural moisturizers. Apply a moisturizer to your skin immediately after bathing if your skin is dry.[4] Adding moisturizer when your skin is still wet will dilute it. Towel dry first, then quickly apply the moisturizer.

SUNSCREEN

I never go out into the sun, so I don't need to wear a sunscreen. I do get in my garden to do some weeding, but I always wear a hat. But I've got this spot on my cheek that just won't heal . . .

—Sophie, age 53

Remember that going out in the sun doesn't necessarily mean lying in the sun. It means carrying on the natural activities of the day that include going to work, going to the grocery store, even sitting in an office under fluorescent lighting.

Sun protection[5] is important for diminishing the risk of skin cancer as well as the risk for unattractive photoaging. A sunscreen of at least sun protective factor (SPF) 15 is important. If you are going to be out in the sun for any length of time, you should use a higher SPF, at least in the 20s or 30s. A hat, sunglasses, and sun-protective clothing are important as well as sunscreen if you are out gardening or elsewhere in the sun for any length of time. Don't forget to protect your eyes. Sun exposure increases the risk of cataracts. Most important, remember to apply and reapply your sunscreen, and see your dermatologist if you have a spot that won't heal.

I've heard that sunscreens need to protect against both UVA and UVB rays. How do I know if my sunscreen has this protection?

—Francis, age 26

Your sunscreen and your sunglasses should protect against ultraviolet A (UVA) rays as well as ultraviolet B (UVB) rays. UVB rays cause sunburn when you stay in the sun too long. Although UVA rays from sunlight don't often cause sunburn, they do penetrate skin deeply and cause damage. UVA rays are found in fluorescent bulbs and some other types of indoor lighting, including lights used in tanning beds.

The label will usually indicate not only the SPF factor but also the type of UV protection. You can also look at the list of ingredients in the sunscreen. Almost all sunscreens protect against UVB, but to see if there is also protection against UVA, look for sunscreen ingredients such as parsol or mexoryl. Sunscreens that contain one or both of these ingredients include Anthelios (La Roche Posay), Hydraphase UV 30 (La Roche Posay), and UV Expert 20 (Lancome). Avobenzone is another ingredient that gives excellent protection against UVA. A major problem with avobenzone, however, is that it does not remain stable for long. Fortunately, technology has now advanced so that a stabilized form of avobenzone has been developed. A patented technology called "helioplex" was utilized by Neutrogena to stabilize avobenzone in combination with oxybenzone, a potent UVB protector, resulting in excellent protection against UVA and UVB. Neutrogena products utilizing the helioplex technology include Ultra Sheer SPF 50+, Ultra Sheer SPF 70, Ultra Sheer SPF 85, and Body Mist SPF 45.

I've been using a tanning bed for the last two months getting ready for my trip to the Bahamas. I don't want to burn on vacation, and the tanning bed has a type of bulb that won't cause skin to burn. But I'm getting these wrinkles around my eyes and on my forehead.

—Susan, age 23

The UVA rays utilized in sun-tanning parlors result in a slow tan and usually do not cause sunburn; but these rays penetrate deeper into the skin—down into the dermis—where damage results. Just because the sun-tanning parlor advertises that you won't burn does not mean that your skin won't be damaged. There's no need to get a tan before your vacation. Use sunscreen or sunblock instead, reapplying it frequently, and wear protective clothing.

I use an SPF of 6 in my makeup. I've heard that all sunscreens are alike, anyway—why should I apply a stronger sunscreen if it's going to be the same as one that I'm using. Besides, those stronger sunscreens feel greasy and smell so strong.
                                                                    —*Brenda, age 19*

No, sunscreens are not all alike. To label a sunscreen with a certain SPF, the manufacturer of the sunscreen must prove to the FDA that the SPF on the label is the true SPF.

How is the SPF of a particular suncreen determined? The amount of sunlight required to cause minimal pinkness of skin in an untanned person is measured. The sunscreen is then applied to another area, and the amount of sunlight necessary to cause minimal pinkness in the area where the sunscreen has been applied is measured. The SPF is calculated from these measurements and tells how much protection the sunscreen gives. For example, it takes 15 times as long to sunburn if a sunscreen with SPF 15 is applied properly.

It is true that you can sweat or swim off your sunscreen. And if you don't reapply, then of course you will lose the protection of the sunscreen. So apply and reapply throughout the day.

What about the greasy feel and odor of sunscreens? Newer, more esthetically acceptable sunscreens with micronized particles are now available. They come in liquids, gels, sprays, and creams and are effective for sun protection, especially if they contain ingredients that protect against UVA rays as well as UVB. Bullfrog, Ombrelle, Antihelios, Solbar, and Neutrogena "Dry Touch" (Ultra Sheer) sunblooks are good sunscreens with UVB and UVA protection, and they don't feel greasy.

My skin always burns and never tans. I heard that sunblocks are the only real way to prevent sun damage. Aren't sunblocks those thick, white creams that lifeguards use? I'd look like a clown wearing that stuff every day!
                                                                    —*Andy, age 17*

Sunblocks block harmful rays from skin by reflecting or scattering light. They present a physical barrier to the entry of the sun rays into skin. Sunscreens, on the other hand, protect skin by absorbing UV radiation. Although sunblocks offer excellent protection against the sun, some are cosmetically unattractive, thick, white creams, such as those used by lifeguards in the sun to protect their noses. Zinc oxide or titanium oxide are common ingredients in sunblocks.

Many sunblocks now, such as the Neutrogena Ultra Sheer sunblocks, come in microsized particles that block sunlight effectively without the white clown look. Whether a good sunscreen or a sunblock is used, fair-skinned persons should be especially careful to also add hats, sunglasses, and protective clothing to protect from the sun.

> *I can't wear sunscreen. The last time I tried to use it, I broke out in a rash all over. It spoiled my vacation at the beach. I'm not doing that again!*
> —Clark, age 19

Some people have a skin sensitivity to certain ingredients in sunscreens. P-aminobenzoic acid (PABA), for example, is very effective protection against UVB, but some people develop redness and itching of skin when using a sunscreen containing PABA. Select your sunscreen well before going on vacation and apply it to one of your arms before applying it all over to make certain that it doesn't cause irritation. If your skin becomes irritated while using a sunscreen, even if it has never caused irritation before, stop using it and change to another sunscreen.

> *I had a great time for the first few days at the beach, and then I got the worst sunburn I've ever had. I don't know what happened. Maybe I didn't reapply my sunscreen after swimming like I should have, but I usually don't burn like this even if I forget to reapply. I was good about remembering to take my acne medications, though.*
> —Ron, age 20

Ron forgot that his doctor said NOT to take his acne medications while at the beach. He was taking tetracycline, an antibiotic that can cause increased sun sensitivity. Certain medications, including oral tetracycline or diuretics that contain thiazides, can cause a blistering reaction of skin to sun exposure. Check with your physician to see if any of your medications are likely to result in increased susceptibility of your skin to sunburn. This can happen with any medication, but the likelihood is higher with certain medications.

> *I feel that a tan makes my skin more attractive. I can't stand that white, sickly look. I feel more healthy with a tan.*
> —Andrea, age 32

Remember that in protecting your skin from the sun, you are not only protecting your skin from damaging radiation that can causes skin cancer, but you are also protecting your skin from photoaging, the most cosmetically damaging and the most preventable form of aging. Tanning will result in skin that looks like tanned leather and a face that looks like a wrinkled prune. If you like the look of a tan but want to avoid sun damage, use the sunless-tanning lotions. Wear that sunscreen! You'll be glad now—and later.

BUILDING UP FROM THE BASICS

If your skin is healthy and young, the more natural the look, the better. Many of us, however, need a little more definition to the eyebrows, to the eyelashes, to the lips, and sometimes a faint blush for the cheeks. A natural hair style—with color touch-up or natural highlights if you wish, good posture, energy, and a confident attitude—and there you have it—a healthy, natural look.

If you have structural skin problems—chin too small or large, unattractive nose—see a plastic surgeon and correct such problems. If you have problems with your complexion—acne, rosacea, dark spots—see a dermatologist and correct these problems. Don't live your life trying to cover up a problem. This often just accentuates it. Fix it!

THE GOLDEN RULE OF SKIN CARE

Try any lotions and creams that you find appealing, but if your skin becomes irritated or if you become unhappy about the appearance of your skin, Go Back to the Basics. By Going Back to the Basics, you will be giving your skin a "rest" from things that can irritate your skin.

By Going Back to the Basics, you will be letting your skin "normalize" in your skin's "Safe Zone." Once your skin is in better shape, you can build your skin care regimen upon the firm foundation of the Basics.

THE GOLDEN RULE

GO BACK TO THE BASICS

CHAPTER 4

SPECIAL CARE FOR HANDS, FEET, NAILS, HAIR, LIPS, AND ELBOWS

E ach of us at one time or another suffers with cracked fingers, sweaty feet, split nails, and dry lips. This chapter will tell you how to care of these problem areas.

CARE OF HANDS AND FEET

I have a terrible problem with my hands. When the weather gets cold, my fingers crack and bleed. Now the weather isn't even cold, and I'm getting them. But I have a new baby, and I'm always changing diapers and washing my hands. What can I do—my hands are so painful!

—Cecilia, age 28

Dry air or contact with harsh substances such as cleaning products can cause hands to crack and bleed—this can indeed be very painful. Irritation of hands and feet is usually worse in winter when the skin is already more dry than in summer. As the furnace is turned up, the heat not only dries your plants, but it also dries your skin. But changing diapers and constantly washing hands can also break down the skin barrier, causing skin to crack and bleed.

Keep a moisturizer next to every sink where you wash your hands, and apply after every hand washing. Dry your hands gently, but dry them well, before applying the moisturizer. During wintertime, it's more important than ever to apply a moisturizer to keep the skin surface from becoming dry. Use a mild, unscented soap such as Dove or Cetaphil for bathing. Pat dry, and quickly apply an unscented moisturizer such as Moisturel Lotion or Eucerin. Feet can become dry, too, so don't forget to apply a moisturizer to your feet after bathing.

Protect your hands when washing dishes by wearing rubber gloves. If the rubber gloves irritate your skin, get thin cotton liners[1] from the drugstore and slip them on before putting on the rubber gloves. If you don't like rubber gloves, use a scrubber with a long handle for washing dishes so that your skin won't have to come in contact with the soapsuds. Soapsuds may feel good to skin, but are murder to the skin barrier.

Some products normally not considered harsh can still irritate your skin if you develop a sensitivity to one of the ingredients in the product. For example, the skin of some individuals is sensitive to antibacterial soap, causing skin irritation. If you are washing your hands a lot, using antibacterial soap, and your fingers are developing painful cracks, change to a mild soap such as Dove.

Some people also develop sensitivity to dyes in clothing. Black or navy hose can irritate legs in some individuals, dark gloves can irritate hands, and dark jersey pullovers can sometimes cause skin to itch. If you are wearing dark clothing and itching, change to light clothing to see if the itching resolves.

> ### TIPS FOR SMOOTH, SOFT HANDS
>
> - Use unscented soap for washing
> - Apply unscented moisturizer
> - Minimize handwashing
> - Wear gloves when washing dishes
> - Avoid coming in contact with harsh substances
> - Apply Vaseline and white cotton gloves overnight to treat rough, chapped hands
> - Tip: Mineral oil and vegetable shortening are good moisturizers for hands

If your fingertips are starting to crack, try applying New Skin liquid bandage (Medtech) or Nexcare liquid bandage drops. Bacitracin ointment to the cracks can also be helpful. If your skin still cracks, see your dermatologist for prescription medication to relieve the problem. Once the cracks have healed, keep a small container or Vaseline or Cetaphil moisturizer with you to apply frequently on fingertips.

> *My feet are a mess. I'm a dedicated runner and just competed in a half-marathon. When I took my running shoes off afterwards, I saw that both my big toes are blue! My feet are sweaty and smell bad, and the skin is cracked and itchy between my toes.*
>
> *—Bryan, age 23*

Jogging can irritate feet and toenails. Shoes that are tight around the toes can cause bruising, especially affecting the large toenails. Bruised toenails may eventually come off, and a new nail grows in. Be sure to wear shoes large enough so that they do not bind around the toes.

Smelly feet can be a sign of infection by a type of bacteria. Your dermatologist may prescribe a topical antibiotic such as erythromycin to treat this condition. White cotton socks or wool socks are best to wear if your feet tend to sweat—nylon or most other synthetic socks won't absorb moisture well. After a long day of work or exercise, put your feet into a tub of warm water—this will make your feet feel wonderful and you will relax. Add a little alcohol or vinegar to the water if your feet are smelly, but not if the skin is cracked, red, or irritated in any way. When bathing, don't forget to wash your feet with soap and rinse well.

Itching and scaling between the toes may be a symptom of athlete's foot, a fungal infection. "Air out" your feet by wearing sandals when possible. Athlete's foot can sometimes be treated with over-the-counter antifungal medication such as Loprox, or you might try soaking your feet in water with a little vinegar added—if your feet are not cracking or bleeding—but if the problem persists, see your dermatologist.

See Chapter 23 for more information on athlete's foot.

The skin on my hands and feet feels thick and rough. I think it's hereditary, because my mother also has thick skin on her hands and feet. Is there anything that I can do to soften them?

—Edith, age 33

If your skin is thick on your hands and feet and you would like to thin and soften it, try AmLactin or Keralyt applied twice a day. Your physician may prescribe LacHydrin Cream[2] (ammonium lactate 12% cream) for this problem. Remember, however, that thick skin may be protective against blistering.

Years ago I spent my summers playing in junior tennis tournaments. I would rest from tennis during the winter, then begin tennis practice again as "tennis season" started in the spring. At the first of the tennis season, I was in misery with painful blisters on my hands and feet from the hours of practice. As summer approached and I practiced more and more, my hands and feet became "toughened." Calluses developed, and no more blisters! I could swing away at the ball knowing that the skin of my hands and feet was now thick enough to protect from blistering. If anyone had offered me a hand cream to soften my hands during those days, I would have thought they were sent by one of my tennis opponents!

CARE OF NAILS

I used to have beautiful nails. Now my fingernails are split at the ends, and my toenails are yellow and thick. What's going on?

—Peggy, age 42

Fingernails and toenails are comprised of layers of keratin, a type of protein. Harsh substances such as fingernail polish remover and detergents can damage nails and cause them to split at the ends. Use protective gloves when washing dishes or using cleaning solutions. Apply a moisturizer or mineral oil to nails after washing hands. Avoid rubbing or nervously picking at your nails or cuticles—this can cause bumpy nails, hangnails, and potential infection. The practice of clipping cuticles is not a good one. Cuticles are there for a purpose—to protect nails. Leave cuticles where they are.

Nails reflect your general health. Certain nail changes can be associated with disorders such as anemia, liver disease, connective tissue disorders, renal failure, and vitamin or mineral deficiency. Thickened yellow or white nails can be a sign of fungal infection. Green nails can signal a bacterial (pseudomonas) infection. Black discoloration of the nail may be a simple bruise, a mole, or a very serious melanoma. See a dermatologist if nail changes occur.

CARE OF HAIR

My scalp is itchy and dry, and my hair seems to be getting thinner, especially in the front. I wear my hair pulled back in a ponytail most of the time—nothing fancy—and I use all the best gels and hair spray to give it body. What am I doing wrong?

—Coleen, age 43

Hair and scalp can become dry from dry air in wintertime, from lack of oil in scalp as you become older, from overtreatment with perms and coloring, or from poor diet or genetic causes.

Wash your hair with a mild shampoo. Use a conditioner after shampooing, if your hair is dry. Avoid frequent permanents, harsh bleach or dyes, hot rollers, or hot hair dryers close to the scalp. Mineral oil rubbed into the scalp at night and washed out in the morning can often remove thick scales on the scalp.

If your scalp is itchy, use a medicated shampoo such as Head and Shoulders and leave on five or ten minutes before rinsing. Wear hair in a natural style—avoid tight ponytails or braids—these can cause you to lose hair, especially around the front hairline.

Avoid using gels, hair spray, and styling mousse as much as possible, since these products often contain perfume, which can irritate skin. Avoid twirling or pulling your hair or scratching your scalp. Eat a balanced diet and get plenty of rest for a healthy scalp. If itchiness and scalp dryness persist, see your dermatologist to check for possible fungal infection of the scalp or other scalp conditions.

CARE OF LIPS

My lips are so dry and chapped that they crack when I smile. I try to keep them moist by licking them, but they just seem to become more and more irritated. What can I do!

—Maureen, age 18

If you lick your lips to try to heal chapped lips and keep them moist, you are only making the condition worse. Licking your lips puts saliva on your lips. Saliva contains enzymes that break down food and can irritate lips. The evaporation of the saliva from your lips will also make your lips dry and irritated.

Use moisturizers, unscented lip balms, or Vaseline to offset lip dryness. A lipstick ingredient may also cause irritation in individuals sensitized to the ingredient. If your lips become easily irritated, use an unscented, hypoallergenic lipstick. Almay has a line of such lipsticks. Avoid lipsticks that you can taste or smell—these are telltale signs of perfume or spices with potential for irritating lips.

Sores around the lips may be "fever blisters" caused by the herpes virus. Such "fever blisters" are infectious and can be transmitted to others through direct contact. Don't kiss anyone if you have a fever blister, and don't share sips from someone's glass or they will share the fever blister too.

See your dermatologist if a problem with irritated lips does not resolve.

THICK SKIN ON ELBOWS

My elbows are the most unattractive part of my body. The skin there looks like alligator skin—rough and thickened. Is there something that will help?
—Barbara, age 33

Elbow skin can dry out and become thickened. Use a moisturizing cream such as Eucerin, Cetaphil Moisturizing Cream, or other mild moisturizers after bathing to keep skin of elbows soft and healthy. Vaseline can be helpful for extremely dry skin.

Over-the-counter AmLactin can also be helpful in smoothing rough skin. Elbows with red, scaling skin can be a sign of psoriasis. If the problem remains, see your dermatologist for evaluation and treatment with prescription medication.

CHAPTER 5

SEVEN SECRETS FOR SENSATIONAL SKIN

I am so busy in my college classes that I haven't taken time to exercise other than walking to the classroom. I've taken an extra course this semester, and term papers are due and finals are coming up. It's all that I can do to get four or five hours of sleep at night. This morning I looked at myself in the mirror and I looked like an old woman!

—*Connie, age 23*

Beautiful skin requires more that taking care of skin alone. Your skin reflects the condition of your body. When you are tired, your skin sags. When you are sick, your skin is pale. When your body is healthy, your skin is first to show your good health.

A HEALTHY BODY

Skin tone improves with rest. Compare how you look at 2 am after a late party with how you look after a good night's sleep. Get the rest that you need—budget your time so that you get at least seven hours of sleep each night! "Power naps" during the day—even for a half an hour if that's all that you can manage—can put you back on your feet with a fresh feeling and fresh skin appearance.

Stay fit. Exercise! Notice how older athletes look much younger than their non-athletic contemporaries. Your circulation delivers oxygen and nutrients to the skin. Exercise improves your circulation

---

SEVEN SECRETS FOR SENSATIONAL SKIN

1. Use a mild soap, a moisturizer if your skin is dry, and a sunscreen
2. Get enough rest—your skin reflects the condition of your body
3. Exercise
4. Eat a balanced diet
5. Don't smoke
6. Reduce stress
7. Be happy; focus on the positive

and overall health of your body, and this is reflected in your skin. Develop an exercise program that you like and can do—make it bicycling or jogging if you like to be outside—or the work-out gym if your time is limited. And stick to the program!

Eat a balanced diet. What we eat affects our skin. Vitamin deficiencies can cause skin problems. Allergies to foods or medicines can cause skin reactions. But be aware that not everyone reacts the same to certain foods. Allergies vary with the individual as well as the severity of skin reaction. Avoid foods that cause problems, and obtain necessary proteins, carbohydrates, minerals, and vitamins from a well-balanced diet so that your body can build strong, healthy skin.

Lean meat and two vegetables, one green and one yellow, add whole grain bread or rice without butter or margarine, fruit for dessert, and you have the ingredients for a healthy meal. If you have a weight problem, take action *now* to lose that weight. Join Weight Watchers or see a nutritionist for help with your diet. Put smaller portions of food on your plate. No nibbling in between meals. When you feel the urge to nibble, pull a bottle of cold water from the refrigerator to drink. Avoid dessert. Avoid white bread, pasta, and other starches. Get out of the house and away from the refrigerator. Be consistent—stick to your diet. Do make sure that you have sufficient protein in your diet—otherwise you'll stay hungry.

Avoid bad habits such as smoking. Smoking deprives your skin of needed oxygen and is bad for your health in other ways. Smoking also contributes to skin aging lines and sagging of skin. As part of the anatomy class in medical school, we had to spend time in the cadaver lab. The lungs of cadavers that had been smokers were black! If you smoke, stop! You'll be much healthier and you'll feel and look like a new person.

Practice stress-reducing exercises. Stress can affect not only your mind but also your skin and the rest of your body. A relaxed, smiling face looks entirely different from a stressed face. Stress can lower the body's ability to resist infection. "Fever blisters," caused by herpes simplex virus, are often precipitated by stress. Acne and eczema can flare during stress. Psoriasis often worsens with stress. Doctors and scientists continue to learn more about the effects of stress on skin. Utilize stress-reduction mechanisms such as massage, meditation, or a quiet corner with a good book, and get plenty of rest.

Take at least two "stress-buster breaks" during the day. Close your eyes, take a deep breath, exhale slowly . . . let your head roll slowly to one side, and then another, then back, then forward. Shake out the tension from your arms and let your arms fall by your side. Tense and then relax each muscle group in turn —first your arms, then your chest, your abdomen, your buttocks, your upper legs, your lower legs, your feet . . . feel the stress leave each muscle group until your body is "dead-weight" . . . Now visualize a quiet beach, waves lapping, blue skies, white sand, seagulls gliding . . . . Even if you set aside only three minutes a day for this, you'll find that it works to reduce stress if you truly block out everything else during that time.

Keep a cheerful outlook. Focus on the positive. You can train yourself to do this even if you do not feel that this is your nature. Your skin reflects your mood. Fright can drain color from your skin; happiness can make your skin flush with healthy color. A happy person has glowing skin. Regardless of your physical appearance, you will be attractive if you have a good attitude, a good sense of humor, and you are happy. Nothing can improve your appearance if you have a bad attitude and are unhappy. Make your cup half full instead of half empty, and you'll be a happier person with more radiant skin.

Stress-Buster Break
1. Close your eyes
2. Take a deep breath
3. Exhale slowly
4. Let your head roll slowly to one side and then to another, then back, and forward
5. Shake your arms and let them fall by your side
6. Tense and then relax each muscle group in turn
7. Take your mind to a quiet place

See your doctor for regular checkups and for treatment of any medical problems. Protecting your health is important for your well-being and for your appearance. You will find that you not only look younger, but you'll feel younger too! Your skin, your body, and your attitude will reflect good care.

A SECRET OF ETERNAL YOUTHFULNESS

On the heels of a divorce from my first husband, I entered law school. The first three months were very stressful, and to eliminate stress and get my body fit for what I then perceived as a three-year nightmare of stress, I started jogging around the university track at 5 am each morning. The first morning that I was on the track, I was jogging in the dark, my eyes fixed on one of the white lines of the track that I could barely see by the glow of a distant streetlight. Suddenly to my fright I heard footsteps running and someone breathing hard behind me. I cowered for the attack, but the footsteps sped by. In the midst of the huffing and puffing, I heard a cheerful call, "Hi Becky!" I was astounded. It was the voice of my 85 year old father. When I was finally able to slow him down after he did four laps, I learned that he ran the track every morning before dawn. Now 97, he no longer runs, but he and my mother, now 90, walk the track each morning and he exercises on the Cybex machines at the YMCA the rest of every morning. There are many reasons why he has maintained his "eternal youthfulness." Among the most important are that (1) He is a happy man who loves life and is excited about every new day and (2) He exercises every single day.

Be excited about life. Each day is a new one to start afresh. Exercise, exercise, exercise. Pick an exercise that you enjoy. If you don't like treadmills, get out and walk. But do something! Every day!

We'll talk in this book about other ways to appear youthful and we'll also talk about what's new on the horizon for reversing signs of aging. First, however, it's important to understand skin—how it looks underneath the surface, and what it does. The next chapter will tell you about your amazing skin.

YOUR AMAZING SKIN

Your skin is miraculous. It does it all. It protects, senses, repairs, regenerates, renews. It is an organ itself, carrying on more than a million different functions and at the same time interacting with the entire body to keep you healthy.

Your skin is your physical barrier between yourself and the environment, protecting you from the outside world, defining your physical boundaries. It stretches and shrinks to accommodate what you and your diet determine to be your physical self.

Skin also protects you in ways that you cannot see. It is an ever-alert sentinel to microscopic invaders that could do harm to your body, sending out its own army of immune cells to attack as necessary.

Skin is also a sensory organ. It lets your body know what is going on around you. Your skin senses whether the outside world is hot, or cold, or wet, or dry. Skin also senses pain or pleasure. Skin sends all of this information to the brain so that the body can adapt as necessary.

Your skin never wears out in performing these protective duties, for it is miraculously capable of renewing itself.

UNDER THE MICROSCOPE

What does skin really look like—up close, under the microscope? First, there is a thin, outer compartment of skin, called the "epidermis." Next, there is a slightly thicker, lower compartment, called the "dermis." Between these two compartments is a "basement membrane." Below the dermis, in the deepest part of skin, is a layer of subcutaneous fat that helps "insulate" us from heat or cold

- Skin is a living organ of many cell layers that are in constant activity.
- These cells communicate with one another and send out signals to coordinate the many skin functions.
- These skin functions include alerting the body's immune system to attempted invasion of skin by bacteria or viruses, repairing wounds, and giving birth to new skin cells.

Figure 6.1. Skin layers. [Courtesy of Blackwell Publishing, Inc. 2004]

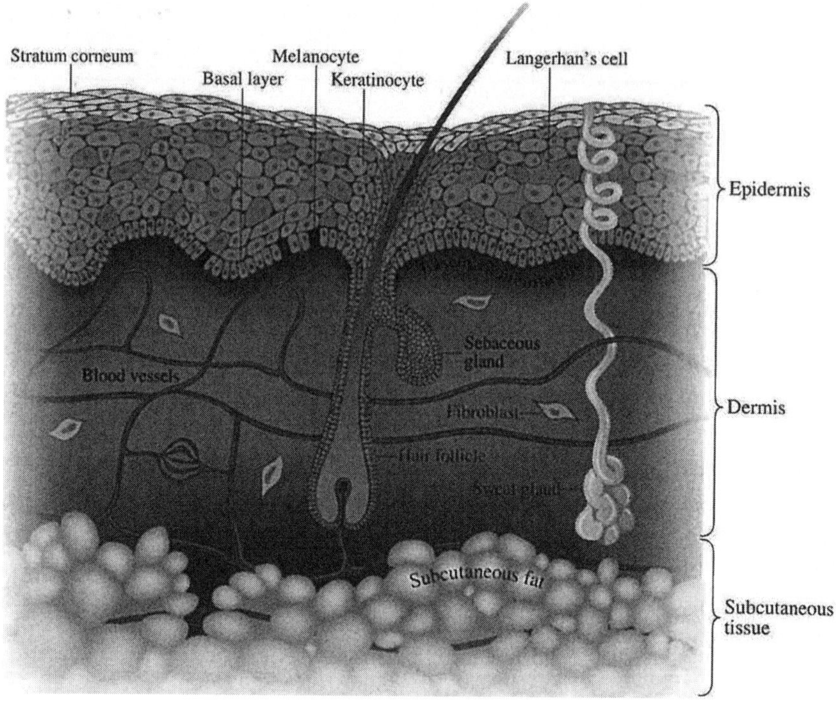

in our environment. Below the layer of subcutaneous fat are muscles, bones, and internal organs. (Figure 6.1)

The Epidermis

Skin cells called "keratinocytes" form the surface of our skin that the world sees. These cells are in constant turnover, with new cells replacing the old cells as cells on the skin surface shed. This shedding is usually not noticed unless skin is flaking and dry, but this process goes on all the time, with continuous renewal of your skin.

Where do the new cells come from that replace the old? They are "born" deep in the *epidermis*, the upper compartment of skin. The epidermis is formed by different layers of keratinocytes. The bottommost layer of the epidermis is the "basal layer." It is here that keratinocytes are "born" and begin their migration to the skin surface to replace the older cells there.

Mother cells, called "stem cells," give birth to the keratinocytes. Unlike the keratinocytes, which migrate to the skin surface, the stem cells remain in the basal layer to give birth to more and more keratinocytes.

The newly-born keratinocytes leave their mother "stem" cells and embark upon a trek upward through many epidermal layers to the skin surface (Figure 6.2). As they move upward through the layers, they are transformed. This process is called "differentiation." In the "spinous layer" of the epidermis, the keratinocytes develop spine-like projections that reach out to touch neighboring keratinocytes. In the "granular layer" they develop internal granules containing powerful enzymes and other substances that they will need to form the protective surface of skin.

As they near the skin surface, the keratinocytes solidify into a "brick and mortar" arrangement like a brick wall. The "mortar" between the bricks is composed mostly of lipids, which help moisturize and protect skin. Finally the keratincytes flatten to form the outer "cornified envelope," the layer that the world sees as our skin.

The life of a keratinocyte as it migrates from the basal layer to the skin surface is only about four weeks, but much is accomplished during that time. As the cells migrate upward they communicate with other keratinocytes to repair wounds, and perform other skin functions. As the new cells move upward to the skin surface, they replace the older cells there. In this way skin constantly renews its surface and provides a competent barrier against wind, weather, and other aspects of the environment.

Although the keratinocytes are the most numerous cells in the epidermis of skin, there are other important cells that reside among the migrating keratinocytes. "Langerhans cells" are immune cells in skin with long projections like spiders with long legs. The Langerhans cells spread out their projections to stand guard for any skin invaders such as bacteria or viruses (Figure 6.3). If an invader makes its way into skin, the Langerhans cells quickly summon help from white blood cells to leave the blood stream and march into skin to attack the invaders. Langerhans cells

Figure 6.2. Just above the basement membrane lies the basal cell layer. It is here that new keratinocytes (skin cells) are born, to begin their upward migration to the surface of skin for skin renewal. [Courtesy of Courtney Vann]

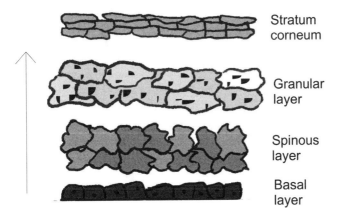

Stratum corneum

Granular layer

Spinous layer

Basal layer

Figure 6.3. The Langerhans cell in the epidermis detects foreign bodies (antigens), captures them, and takes them to immune cells in the lymph nodes for elimination. Tennis racket-shaped Birbeck granules are seen in Langerhans cells. Their function is not clear. [Courtesy of Courtney Vann]

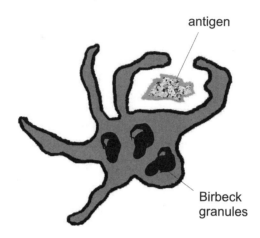

also alert the white blood cell army to damaged skin cells that must be disposed of before they can cause problems.

"Melanocytes" also live in the epidermis. They are most often found in the basal layer among the stem cells (Figure 6.4). These cells produce dark pigment (tan)

Figure 6.4. Melanocytes produce pigment to transfer to keratinocytes in little packets called melanosomes. The transferred pigment produces the color of our skin. [Courtesy of Courtney Vann]

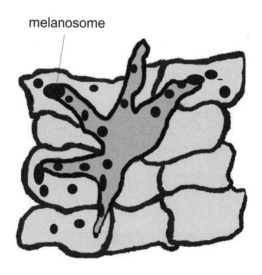

when exposed to sun. This pigment fans out in the skin layers to screen our skin from the bright sun rays. This helps protect our skin cells from sun damage. At first glance this would seem to imply that sun tanning is good. But the sun's rays can still penetrate skin and do damage to all skin cells, including the dark melanocytes. While a tan can be somewhat protective, damage to cells can still occur, resulting in skin cancers and photoaging. It is best to wear sunscreen and protective clothing.

Nerve cells also live in the epidermis. Each has a different function. One type senses pressure; another type senses heat or cold; still another type senses vibration.

These cells send signals to the brain to give information about what is going on in the body's environment so that the body can respond accordingly.

Working together, the cells of the epidermis coordinate with each other to repair, renew, and protect.

The Basement Membrane

Below the basal layer of the epidermis is the "basement membrane." This is a protective layer that separates the epidermis from the "dermis," the lower compartment of skin. This layer also serves to attach the epidermis to the dermis through proteins that assemble into an "anchoring complex." This anchoring complex attaches to the basal layer of the epidermis and extends down into the dermis. In certain conditions, defects in the basement membrane cause skin to "blister off," emphasizing the importance of this layer.

The Dermis

Deep in skin, below the basement membrane, lies the *dermis*, the lower compartment of skin. Important activities are in progress here also.

Figure 6.5. Fibroblasts in the dermis produce collagen and elastin for skin firmness and elasticity. [Courtesy of Courtney Vann]

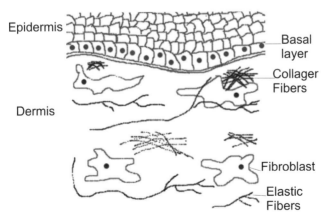

The dermis is the true foundation for our skin. Here are the collagens and elastins that give our skin firmness and elasticity. The main cells in the dermis are "fibroblasts," which produce collagen and elastin. These substances not only contribute to a youthful appearance to skin but also are important in wound repair for deeper skin injuries (Figure 6.5).

The epidermis does not contain blood vessels. It is therefore dependent upon nutrients from blood vessels in the dermis. While the epidermis prevents loss of moisture from skin, the dermis and the subcutaneous fat below the epidermis give structure to skin and help insulate the body, providing a buffer to cold and heat in the environment.

SKIN CELLS AND THEIR WORLD OF COMMUNICATION

In order to perform important skin functions, skin cells must communicate and act in a coordinated manner. Skin cells communicate by secreting substances called "cytokines." The cytokines provide signals that produce other signals that interact and cascade with other cell signals in a beautifully complex orchestration

Figure 6.6. When an antigen invades skin, a signal cascade results that calls immune cells to attack and instructs skin to repair itself. [Courtesy of Rebecca Campen, M.D.]

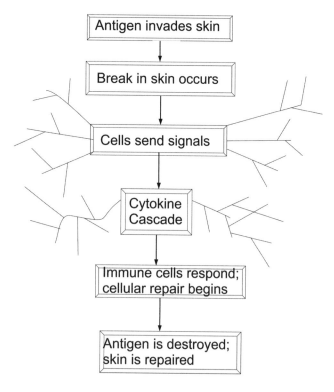

that results in wound healing, skin renewal and other skin functions (Figure 6.6). Each cell has receptors on its surface, like antennae, that recognize and interpret the cytokine messages sent.

Scientists continue to marvel at what our skin cells do in their microscopic world. The beauty of our universe is indeed much more than we can see.

CHAPTER 7

WHEN SKIN AGES: THE SCIENTIFIC BASIS

It happens to all of us. Our skin ages as the rest of our body ages. But what really happens when skin ages?

We all know what aging looks like on the skin surface. Skin becomes drier, complexion more sallow, skin sags, and blood vessels become more prominent. Blood vessels may rupture more easily, causing dark purple bruises, especially on the arms. Hair becomes more sparse, and bald spots may appear, especially on men's scalps.

But what happens *inside* skin with aging?

First, the top layer of skin, the epidermis, becomes thinner, thus affording less "barrier" protection from the outside world. For skin to "work well," it needs this "barrier" protection. A thinner epidermis means that moisture is lost more easily through skin, and skin often becomes dry and flaky. As skin is exposed to sun and other elements of our environment, cells become damaged and can multiply uncontrollably, giving rise to skin cancers and other problems.

Second, immune cells in skin become less efficient in seeking out and eliminating damaged cells. This allows some damaged cells that can cause skin cancer to go undetected.

Third, pigment cells (melanocytes) in the epidermis begin to work less effectively. Sun exposure results in dark spots and spotches, even in people who tanned evenly at an earlier age.

Fourth, fibroblasts in the dermis work less efficiently. Remember that these are the cells in the dermis that produce collagen and elastin. Collagen gives shape and structure to skin. As fibroblasts produce less collagen, the skin becomes less firm, and wrinkles form. Elastin gives elasticity to skin. Fibroblasts try hard to keep up production of elastin, but many elastin fibers are fragmented, "clogging up the works" rather than providing good elasticity to skin. As production of normal elastin falls, skin sags.

Fifth, certain important hormones such as estrogen, testosterone, dehydroepiandrosterone sulfate (DHEAS), and growth hormone decrease. Hormones affect all skin functions, and when they decrease with aging, skin firmness and elasticity are adversely affected.

Sixth, muscles underlying skin become weaker, and muscle tone is more lax. In young skin, muscles compete with other muscles to keep skin smooth and tight, just as two hands each pulling opposite ways on a cloth keep the cloth smooth and tight. When muscles become weaker and cannot keep up such competition, deep wrinkles can occur.

Seventh, hair follicles, sweat glands, and sebaceous glands do not work as efficiently with aging. Hair keeps us warm. Sweat glands produce sweat to cool the body. Sebaceous glands contribute lipids to the surface of skin to moisturize[1] and to enhance skin barrier protection. With aging, hair follicles become smaller ("miniaturization") and hair thins. Sweat glands work less effectively, and the body may feel too warm or too cold. Sebaceous glands do not work as efficiently to provide lipids to the skin surface, and skin becomes dry.

All of these things happen with *intrinsic* skin aging. That is, with the "ticking clock" that is internal to all of us. The hands of time move forward, and there's no way to halt them or make them move backward. But there is a form of aging that *can* be stopped. We'll talk more about this in a minute.

What about antiwrinkle creams that we see advertised? It is important to remember the structure of skin and to understand that any treatment that *really* treats wrinkles at its source must reach down into the dermis, the deeper layer of skin, to stimulate the fibroblasts to produce more collagen and elastin. Creams alone *just don't get down this far into skin*. While antiwrinkle creams won't cure wrinkles, they *can* act as moisturizers to keep the skin surface smooth. With such creams, tiny superficial wrinkles may be less noticeable, just as with use of any moisturizer, but deeper wrinkles won't be affected.

The really good news is that effective treatment of wrinkles is the Number-One Priority of most skin care companies that are collaborating with scientists. Chapter 29 will give a peek at what's in store for treating wrinkles in the not-too-distant future.

If we can't turn back the clock to stop intrinsic aging, is there anything that we can do to correct some of the things that are happening? Is there any way to make us look younger? The answer is yes. In Chapter 8 we'll look at some of the treatments that can have a dramatic effect on signs of skin aging.

A REVERSIBLE CAUSE OF SKIN AGING

I know now that sun isn't good for your skin, but I grew up in ing on baby oil and lying in the sun. We thought tanning was a healthy thing then. I even remember using aluminum foil to try to reflect more rays and get a tan sooner. Now I'm paying the price—my face looks like a dried-up prune!

—Alicia, age 53

Although there is no way yet to prevent *intrinsic* skin aging, *extrinsic* skin aging is another story. *Extrinsic* skin aging is just what the name implies—caused by factors outside of the body. Such factors in the environment include wind, cold, and *especially* sun exposure. You *can* do something about this form of skin aging.

Sun exposure causes a premature form of skin aging that is *preventable*. Skin aging that results from sun exposure is called "photoaging." Think about this when you are considering tanning. You may get a tan, but your skin will age *prematurely*, and that's not a pretty picture. There are many people like Alicia whose skin now looks like a dried-up prune because of tanning.

Don't be misled that a tanning booth is safe for your skin. The tanning parlor may claim that you'll tan, not burn, because of special types of bulbs that are used. Most tanning booths do indeed use UVA irradiation, which results in less burning than UVB irradiation. But this does *not* mean that your skin won't be damaged. UVA rays penetrate *deeper* into the skin than UVB rays. You will be damaging the very collagens and elastin in the dermis that give your skin its firmness. Your skin will sag and wrinkle and you'll look old.

With sun exposure, normal flow of signals between the epidermis and dermis is disrupted. Langerhans cells, those important immune cells in the epidermis, become sluggish in trying to respond to antigen challenge, and the likelihood of skin cancers is increased.

Many keratinocytes are damaged and can die or worse, become cancerous. Stem cells in the basal layer of the epidermis are compromised, resulting in less efficient skin turnover to replace damaged cells, and therefore skin "renewal" is compromised.

Sun exposure also causes fragmentation of elastic fibers, a double whammy to the already-reduced quantity of elastic fibers because of intrinsic aging. Severe skin wrinkling and sagging can result. The basement membrane, like the elastic fibers, begins to fragment. As the basement membrane begins to fragment, the body tries to repair it, resulting in "reduplication" of the basement membrane.

Remember that "tanning" is the process used to change skin into leather. To prevent premature aging from sun exposure, protect your skin from the sun. Wear hats and sunglasses and apply sunscreen.

Although there's no magic breakthrough yet in reversing *intrinsic* aging, you *can* prevent *extrinsic* aging caused by photoaging. This is the most obvious and unattractive form of aging, so wear that sunscreen!

If the damage is already done, and your skin is wrinkled from years in the sun, is there anything that you can do to restore a youthful appearance?

Absolutely.

The next chapters will tell you how to look and feel young again.

CHAPTER 8

AMAZING TRANSFORMATIONS
IN YOUR APPEARANCE

I grew up in California and spent most of my free time on the beach. I've learned my lesson now about the damage that the sun can do—look at these creases in my face! So now I wear a sunscreen and do my walking early in the morning or late in the afternoon. But is there anything that I can do about these wrinkles! I have my 20th college reunion coming up and I just can't face everybody like this!

—*Mary Ann, age 44*

As we age, our skin sags and wrinkles and its color becomes sallow and mottled. Hair becomes thinner, and leg veins become more prominent. Unwanted skin growths occur, along with dry skin and itching. Treating these problems can create a much more positive outlook on life as well as a more youthful appearance.

If you are dreading your reunion or just eager to rediscover your youthful appearance, there's hope. Never before have there been so many cosmetic procedures that can dramatically erase signs of skin aging.

BOTOX, FACIAL RESURFACING, CHEMICAL PEELS, AND MORE

There are chemical peels to stimulate skin turnover and renewal. There are deeper peels, dermabrasion, and laser resurfacing to reduce wrinkles and smooth skin. Liposuction can resculpture the body, removing unwanted fat from abdomen, thighs, neck, and other areas. Tissue augmentation and fat transfer can fill in wrinkles, make cheekbones and chin more prominent, and lips more full and defined. Facelifts can tighten skin and reduce years from your appearance. Botox can relax wrinkles and smooth furrowed brows.

We'll talk about these techniques in this chapter. It is important to understand not only the potential benefits, but also the potential side effects of any procedure that you contemplate. Make sure that the dermatologist or plastic surgeon that will be performing the procedures is board certified has had a lot of experience doing the procedures.

SCLEROTHERAPY

I can't go swimming or wear shorts anymore. I have these awful leg veins that make my legs look awful! I don't even like to wear skirts because these veins are also around my ankles. I've heard there are lasers now that can treat these. Is this true?

—Melinda, age 30

"Sclerotherapy,"[1] rather than laser treatment, is best for treatment of superficial leg veins, although lasers are in development that may soon be useful for this kind of treatment. When sclerotherapy is performed, the doctor injects a small amount of solution (hypertonic saline or sodium tetradecyl sulfate [STS, Sotradecol]), into the unwanted veins. The solution disrupts the vein walls and the vein usually disintegrates over the next two or three weeks. Not all veins go away with the first treatment. Follow-up treatment will often be necessary to treat those veins that did not respond the first time.

Sometimes one injection will affect several connected veins, so it is not always necessary to inject separately every single vein. There may be some minor discomfort (some stinging and mild cramping of legs) with the injections. There is sometimes bruising that usually goes away in several weeks. There also may be tiny scars at the sites of injection.

After treatment the doctor may apply cotton balls and tape to the injection sites, and your legs may be wrapped with ace wraps to hold the cotton balls in place. You will probably be asked to wear support stockings for two or three weeks to help get rid of the veins that have been treated. You may want to wait until cool weather before having this procedure—support hose can be very hot in the summertime!

Good technique is very important. Be sure that your dermatologist has performed a lot of sclerotherapy.

Is the solution that is injected safe?

Hypertonic saline is a sterile, concentrated salt solution. Allergic reactions do not usually occur to this solution unless there is allergy to a preservative in the saline. Allergic reactions to Sotradecol rarely occur. Discuss the procedure and potential side effects with your dermatologist prior to treatment.

What about varicose (bulging) veins? Can they be treated?

Varicose (bulging) veins are not usually treated with sclerotherapy, but they can be removed surgically by vascular surgeons and dermatological surgeons that perform this procedure.

Can I resume regular activities after sclerotherapy?

You can usually continue your regular activities after sclerotherapy as long as there is no discomfort or cramping.

FACIAL PEELS[2]

I felt like my skin needed something to "pick it up". My skin felt rough and I had these dark spots on my cheeks that appeared when I was taking birth control pills and sunbathing. I don't know what I need—just something not too harsh—but something that will make my face look "fresh" again.

—Sandra, age 29

Facial peels are cosmetic procedures that temporarily improve the surface of skin. There are "superficial peels," "medium depth peels," and "deep peels," depending upon how far down into the skin the effects will occur. The deeper the peel, the more dramatic the cosmetic effect, but the longer the recovery time.

Superficial Peels

Superficial peels are sometimes called "lunchtime peels" because the side effects are usually mild, with temporary pinkness and mild skin irritation. These peels smooth the skin by clearing dead skin away from the skin surface, allowing a fresh, new surface to generate. These peels also treat some types of acne and can lighten some dark spots on the face. They do not, however, significantly affect facial wrinkling or other signs of skin aging.

What happens when you have a superficial peel? An aesthetician in a doctor's office often performs a superficial peel after the doctor's initial exam. You will wash your face in the doctor's office to remove makeup. The aesthetician will then apply a mild acid to your face. The acid is usually an alpha hydroxyl acid (e.g., glycolic acid) or a beta hydroxyl acid (e.g., salicylic acid). The acid will be left on your face for several minutes. There may be some mild stinging and burning and you may be given a little hand-held fan to cool your face. The acid will then be neutralized, and your face washed clean of the acid. You will be instructed to apply sunscreen to protect your face from the sun.

Usually a series of peels will be done over the next several weeks, with the strength of acid increased each time as possible. After this initial series, the doctor may recommend that you have a "maintenance" facial peel every two or three months to maintain your new "fresh" look.

Medium Depth Peels

Medium depth peels require a slightly longer convalescent time, and there is greater risk for some scarring and skin color changes. Medium strength acids, such as Jessner's Solution or trichloroacetic acid,[3] are used. These acids remove more skin than mild acids and have more of an effect on the signs of aging. Medium depth peels can be useful in treating some precancers (actinic keratoses) and in treating acne, superficial wrinkling, and some types of color changes in skin from sun exposure. More skin peeling and redness occurs with these medium depth peels than with superficial peels.

Deep Peels

Deeper peels, such as phenol peels or those using strong concentrations of tricholoracetic acid, affect deep layers of the skin as well as the medium and superficial layers. These peels treat mottling of skin color from sun exposure as well as superficial and deep wrinkles. More skin is removed from the upper layer of skin (epidermis), stimulating regeneration of a new upper layer. Depending upon the strength of the acid, the lower part of skin (dermis) may also be stimulated to produce more collagen and elastin, making more collagen and reducing wrinkles.

Deep peels have a longer convalescent time—sometimes three to six weeks or more. There is also increased risk of scarring and increased risk that your skin will develop light or dark patches where treated.

There may be other potential side effects. If you are interested in having a facial peel, see a dermatologist or plastic surgeon for an evaluation to determine whether you are a candidate and what type of peel would be best for you. Be sure to tell the doctor if you have a tendency to form large scars, if you have had cold sores, or if you have any other medical problems. This is important information in determining whether a peel would be a suitable choice for you. Always ask about potential side effects of any peel that is determined suitable for you.

WHAT ABOUT FACIALS?

Facials usually include massage, application of hot towels, and application of various creams, lotions, "natural products," astringents, and other substances. They feel wonderful and help you relax, and the stress reduction that can come from such relaxation can be a great benefit.

But that's about as far as the benefit goes—facials are not particularly therapeutic for skin care. In fact, you want to avoid facials if you have acne. Sebaceous gland activity can be stimulated by facial massage, causing acne to flare. If you like facials and haven't had any problems, go ahead and enjoy them. But avoid them if your face becomes irritated or acne develops.

DERMABRASION

I had really bad acne during my teen years. Now that I'm in my 30's I don't have acne any more, but I have all of these acne scars all over my face. Is there anything that I can do?

—Randy, age 35

Dermabrasion[4] is a technique used to "sand down" the skin to remove scars and blemishes. A special "sanding tool" is used to remove the upper layer (epidermis) of skin. Skin alone is too soft to sand well, so fluid is injected into the area to be sanded (the skin is made "tumescent"), or the area is cooled so that it becomes frozen and more stiff. The skin is then "sanded" with a dermabrasion instrument until the upper layer of skin is removed. Dermabrasion can "resurface" skin by eliminating superficial wrinkles and can diminish acne scars.

Depending upon how much "sanding" is done, some medium depth wrinkles can also be diminished. Too much sanding, however, can result in scarring, so deeper acne scars and deeper wrinkles are best treated by other means, such as by injection of Restylane or other filler substances discussed later in this chapter.

After dermabrasion there is usually a recovery time of at least three to six weeks.

MICRODERMABRASION

Dan's taking me out to dinner this weekend when he's back in town. I think this may turn out to be a very special evening. I wish I could do something about my face to make it smoother, to make my skin look better, without doing anything drastic. Is there anything that I can do that will help without making me look like a freak this weekend? This is a really important date!
—*Samantha, age 25*

Microdermabrasion is a more gentle form of removing skin than dermabrasion. This procedure can improve sun-damaged skin of face, neck, and hands; improve acne; and diminish fine wrinkling.

The skin is "lightly sanded" with a pressure stream of microsized particles such as aluminum oxide crystals or with other "light sanding" means. It is not necessary to inject the skin with fluids or freeze it to make it stiff, as is necessary with dermabrasion.

Microdermabrasion usually removes less epidermis than dermabrasion and normally requires little to no recovery time. Although the results will not be as dramatic as with dermabrasion, the results can be pleasing with smoother, silkier skin. Normally only part of the epidermis is removed, but the number of times the same area is treated in a session will determine how deep in skin the treatment reaches.

Appropriate treatment is less irritating than most other skin-resurfacing techniques, but overly-aggressive treatment can result in persistent pinkness of skin, changes in skin color, and scarring.

LASER ABLATION OF VASCULAR LESIONS

I've got this red spider-like spot right on the tip of my nose that appeared while I was pregnant—and there's another one on my right cheek. And I've got red spots appearing all over my stomach now. I'm so self-conscious, especially about the ones on my face—makeup just doesn't cover them. What can I do?
—*Celia, age 35*

Cherry angiomas are tiny red bumps comprised of blood vessel cells. They may be found on the chest, abdomen, back, or any other areas of skin. Facial telangectasia are spider-like blood vessels on the face. These growths are not harmful, but many people don't want them, especially if they are on the face. They can usually be removed ("ablated") in the doctor's office by laser[5] or by electrocautery using a fine needle.

Side effects of laser treatment of these "vascular" growths (made of blood vessel or blood vessel components) include bruising that normally fades during the next several weeks. Sometimes these spots regrow over time and may need to be treated again.

Port wine stains (big purple/red birthmarks sometimes seen on the face) and hemangiomas (red or pink spots or growths) are also vascular and can be treated with laser. Many treatments may be necessary for significant improvement of port wine stains and hemangiomas. Large spots may not totally go away, but results can be dramatic in some cases.

Some hemangiomas that appear on babies at birth will go away on their own over time; others will not. If your baby has a hemangioma, ask your child's pediatrician if it is the type that will eventually go away or if it is not likely to do so. He or she can refer you to a specialist for treatment of the lesion if the pediatrician thinks that is necessary.

LASER RESURFACING

I've been a tennis player all of my life and haven't been good about applying sunscreen. I'm 35 now and my skin looks like I'm 80. Is there any way that I can just get a whole new face?

—Elizabeth, age 35

Laser resurfacing[6] is a technique to remove wrinkles, "tighten" facial skin, and generate "new skin." A high-energy laser[7] is used to burn off the epidermis of facial skin. This not only stimulates the epidermis to regenerate new skin but also causes the dermis to produce new collagen and elastin important in keeping skin firm and supple and preventing or eliminating wrinkles.

There can be dramatic results with laser resurfacing, especially on photoaged skin. Dark spots can fade and small wrinkles can disappear as skin tightens slightly from the process. Scars from acne can also be diminished.

Basically what happens is that the skin is, indeed, resurfaced. The top layer of old skin is burned off bit by bit with the laser, wiped clean from the face, and a new top layer is allowed to grow. The process would be painful without anesthesia, so local or general anesthesia is used.

Ointment is applied to the treatment area, and a dressing that usually covers all of the face except the eyes, nose, and mouth, is applied. An average of 4–6 weeks is usually needed for recovery. Side effects can occur as long as six or seven months after the procedure and can include skin irritation, patchy loss or darkening of skin color, scarring, infection, acne, or other complications.

Although laser skin resurfacing is used primarily for facial skin resurfacing, this technique can be applied to the neck, hands, and arms with some improvement of wrinkles and mottled pigmentation, but scarring and discoloration can result in these areas also.

Discuss the pros and cons of treatment with your dermatologist or plastic surgeon. Be sure to tell your doctor if you have ever had cold sores, a history of collagen vascular disease or other immune disorders, or if you have a tendency to form keloids or hypertrophic scars. This information is important for determining if you are a candidate for this procedure. Isotretinoin and some other types of medications should not be taken during the treatment period.

INTENSE PULSED LIGHT (IPL) TREATMENT

My daughter is getting married in two months, and I really want to firm up my skin and get rid of these wrinkles, but I just can't take the time off from work that my doctor says I would need to have a deep chemical peel or laser resurfacing. Isn't there any other way?

—Rachael, age 52

Up until now the procedures that we have discussed that really do something about wrinkles have required sanding, burning, or chemical peeling the skin. But the fast-paced life style that we live has demanded something less damaging to the surface of skin that will affect the deeper layers of skin where the secret to treating wrinkles lies.

The answer was developed based on research at the Wellman Center of Photomedicine at the Massachusetts General Hospital. Inspired by this research, an IPL treatment was developed that does not burn off the epidermis, but instead penetrates down into the dermis to stimulate fibroblasts to make new collagen and elastin that give support and firmness to skin (Palomar Star Lux IPL System). Other industries have now developed IPL systems based on similar concepts.

With most IPL therapies there can be improvement in skin tone and texture, reduction in mild wrinkles, reduction of scars from acne, and elimination of tiny blood vessels on the face. Some color changes in skin, such as dark circles under the eyes, can also be reduced.

Although the results of IPL treatment are not as dramatic or as long-lasting as laser resurfacing, and tightening of skin and wrinkle reduction will not be as dramatic, there are fewer complications, and the recovery time is much shorter.

"Fraxel" is a popular new treatment also developed from research at the Wellman Laboratories of Photomedicine. A grid-like arrangement of laser beams results in millions of tiny "columns" of skin, leaving tiny areas of untreated skin in between. The treated "columns" shrink, acting like millions of tiny mini-facelifts, tightening skin evenly across the face.

As with any other cosmetic procedure, discuss potential side effects as well as benefits with your physician.

LIPOSUCTION

I'm so frustrated by my attempts to lose weight. I've gone on every kind of diet, and although I've lost lots of pounds, nothing that I do seems to get rid of this fat on my thighs!

—Patricia, age 34

Liposuction[8] may be able to suction away that fat. Liposuction is NOT the answer to losing weight. Diet and exercise are the best way to try to lose weight. But liposuction can be the answer to removing certain fat deposits to "sculpture" the body. This procedure can remove fat from thighs, abdomen, hips, upper arms, the chin, neck, and any other areas with unwanted fat.

How does liposuction work? As you lie on a procedure table, the doctor inserts long metal instrument (cannula), like a tiny vacuum hose, into the fat and moves it back and forth, breaking up fat and sucking the residue into a container. A vacuum in the tip of the instrument provides the suction. Following the procedure, pressure bandages are applied. There will be some bruising and some discomfort. Recovery time is a couple of weeks. Be sure that the physician performing the procedure has much experience in this area. There have been a few deaths from liposuction where too much fat was removed at one time.

Remember, it is best to achieve your desired weight *before* you have liposuction. It is important to keep weight off after the procedure also, as fat will accumulate in the non-liposuctioned areas. Discuss the procedure and potential side effects with your dermatologist or plastic surgeon if you are considering liposuction.

TISSUE AUGMENTATION

I've given up. I'm accepting that I'm old. My lipstick won't go on right anymore—there's no defined line to my lips anymore—and my cheeks have sagged. It's all over!

—Anne, age 63

Anne could benefit by a technique called "tissue augmentation" to give her renewed hope and a youthful look. Tissue augmentation[9] adds substance and definition to certain skin areas.

A receding chin, for example, can be "filled in" with various substances so that it is attractively prominent rather than receding. Cheek bones and lips can be better defined, and wrinkles can be "filled in" so that they seem to disappear. Various substances can be injected to achieve these effects.

Different types of collagen, such as Zyderm-I,[10] Zyderm-II[11], and Zyplast,[12] can be implanted (injected) under the skin to smooth away wrinkles and scars. These collagens are derived from purified cow collagen, and each type serves a slightly different purpose. Zyderm-I implants are used to treat fine wrinkles and shallow scars, "crows feet," and nasolabial (between nose and lips) lines of the face. Zyderm-II implants are used to treat moderate wrinkles and scars. Zyplast implants are used to treat deeper wrinkles and scars, nasolabial lines, and to better define lip borders. AlloDerm,[13] collagen derived from human cadavers, is also used to treat wrinkles and scars.

Collagen injections are done in the office, and most patients can return to their normal activities after the procedure. The results usually last from three to six months before the collagen is absorbed by the body. Since some people may have an allergic reaction to the cow collagen with temporary redness and swelling of the injected site, a skin test is performed on the forearm and observed for three to four weeks before other areas are treated. Because AlloDerm is human collagen, there is less chance of allergic reaction than with cow collagen, but a skin test should still be done.

CosmoDerm is a human bioengineered collagen for treatment of the little "smokers' lines" above the upper lip. CosmoPlast is a human bioengineered collagen for giving definition to the lip outlines to keep lipstick from "bleeding" outward from the lips. Since these are human collagens, they do not require skin testing prior to use.

One's own fat can also be used for tissue augmentation. This is called "micro lipoinjection."[14] The fat is "harvested" by liposuction of a fatty area, such as the buttock, and then the fat is injected wherever augmentation is desired, such as in wrinkles of the face, acne scars, or to make the chin or cheeks more prominent.

Recently hyaluronic acid (Restylane, Juvederm) has become a popular substance for tissue augmentation. Hyaluronic acid is a substance normally found in human skin and helps give "structure" to skin. Hyaluronic acid used in tissue augmentation was originally obtained from rooster combs, which contain a lot of this substance. Most present day hyaluronic acid used for tissue augmentation is bioengineered.

The injectable hyaluronic acids can also be used to increase lip size.[15] Since lip injections can be painful, a "dental block" with lidocaine is often given prior to the injections. This involves injections into the gum tissue to numb the areas to be injected. Some recent new hyaluronic acid injectable substances are incorporating lidocaine to decrease discomfort during injection.

Hands are often the most prominent "give away" sign of aging, with thinning, sagging skin and blue veins just under the skin surface. Although tissue augmentation is most frequently used to "sculpture" facial skin, it can also be used to minimize the appearance of prominent veins on hands and to give a smoother, more youthful appearance to the hands. Side effects can include bruising and swelling as well as unevenness of the skin surface.

HAIR TRANSPLANTATION

I started losing hair around my temples when I was in my early twenties. I knew it would happen—there are lots of other balding men in my family. Now my hairline starts way back on my head, and I try to keep my hair long enough to comb it over the bald areas—but as soon as the wind blows, it's all over. I've heard that hair transplantation has improved to the point that it's hard to tell it's been done.

—Mickey, age 45

Hair transplantation[16] restores hair to bald areas of the scalp or where hair is thinning. You may have noticed that even in people that are bald on top of the head, many seem to keep growing hair around the lower back of the scalp. In hair transplantation this area at the back of the scalp is used to obtain hair follicles to implant into bald areas.

The doctor surgically excises a long strip of scalp from the posterior scalp, along with the hair from that area. The doctor's technicians dissect hair follicles ("minigrafts") from this strip of scalp while the doctor makes tiny stab cuts into the bald areas for implantation of the minigrafts.

In the "old days" of hair transplantation, larger "plugs" of tissue containing hairs were placed into cuts into the scalp instead of minigrafts. The scars that resulted after transplantation of these plugs made it obvious that hair transplantation had occurred. Todays minigrafts result in a much more natural look.

Hair transplantation usually requires several "sessions" and full effects won't be evident for about six months, but results can be dramatic.

SCALP REDUCTION

I've got just one round bald spot about the size of a silver dollar on my scalp. Can't you just cut it out?

—Andrew, age 42

Yes. Scalp reduction may be the answer for Andrew. This means cutting out the bald spots and sewing the scalp together to repair the cut area so that the areas where hair is still growing will be close together rather than separated by bald areas. This can give a dramatic appearance of new hair growth. As much of the bald area as possible is removed, and patches of thinning hair that may be left, or that may develop later, can be "filled in" by hair transplantation. If the bald area is too large to excise completely, the scalp around the area to be excised can be "expanded" by surgically implanting something like a balloon under the scalp and inflating it a little bit each day until more skin is forced to grow, resulting in more scalp tissue to close the area after excision. Even though the bald area is excised, Andrew can still continue to lose hair in this area over time. Another option for Andrew is finasteride (Propecia[17]), discussed further in Chapter 17.

BLEPHLAROPLASTY

My upper eyelids have sagged so much that they almost hang over my eyes when I'm tired. And my lower lids sag like I've got bags hanging there. Is there anything that I can do to make my eyes look young again?

—*Leigh Anne, age 37*

Blephlaroplasty[18] lifts the skin of your upper and lower eyelids by removing fat and excess skin from these areas. This procedure can be combined with other types of skin lifts to erase years from one's appearance.

Side effects include bruising and discloration around the eyes that can last for about two weeks.

Blephlaroplasty is performed by plastic surgeons, oculoplastic surgeons, and some cosmetic dermatologists and can give dramatic results in reversing the appearance of sagging lids and bags under the eyes.

OTHER SKIN LIFTS

I'm 65 years old and have had the luxury of spending much of my life outdoors playing tennis and golf. At one time I thought this was great for my skin—I always had a tan—but now I envy my friends who had to work all of their life. They haven't spent their lives in the sun like I have, and their skin is still smooth and relatively wrinkle-free. But look at my skin—it folds and wrinkles all over itself. I feel like a 90 year old. Would some of these new treatments that I hear about help me?

—*Mary Anne, age 65*

A face lift is the answer here. The full facial skin lift is the most effective way to restore a more youthful appearance to a sagging and heavily wrinkled face.

There are also "partial" face lifts where parts of the face, including earlobes, lips, and neck, are lifted. Lip lifts can make lips appear fuller and eliminate sagging at the corners of the mouth. Excess skin removed from the neck, under the chin, or under the eyes, can result in a more youthful appearance. See a plastic surgeon for discussion of different types of skin lifts of other surgical corrections that can dramatically affect how you look. Be sure to ask about side effects and "down time" for recovery.

Mary Anne may also need some facial resurfacing in some areas in conjunction with the face lift.

HAIR REMOVAL

I've got this dark hair above my lips in the moustache area that is so embarrassing. When I bleach it, it looks orange. I tried electrolysis, but my skin became irritated. Could the new laser hair removal techniques that I've heard about help?

—Barbara, age 35

Unwanted hair can often be eliminated with electrolysis[19] or with laser treatment,[20] both of which destroy the hair follicle. Laser hair removal works best on dark hairs since the laser usually targets the melanin (dark color) in hair. Non-ablative lasers (intense pulsed light) can also remove dark hair. Several treatments may be necessary, and some hair may regrow. Blond, red, or gray hairs do not respond well to laser or intense pulsed light hair removal. Electrolysis is an option for removal of light-colored hairs.

Vaniqa[21] (eflornithine hydrochloride) is a prescription cream that slows the rate of facial hair growth. It can be used in combination with methods that remove hair such as electrolysis and laser hair removal. If you are plucking remaining hairs, you won't have to pluck as often if Vaniqa is applied regularly to the area.

If you are interested in laser hair removal, discuss the procedure with your dermatologist.

WRINKLE REDUCTION

I don't want any procedures that will make me have to take time off from work and cost a fortune. Isn't there any cream that will do something about these wrinkles?

—Diane, age 42

Much money is spent by consumers on creams and treatments to remove wrinkles. But are they effective? Does any cream really remove wrinkles?

Renova[22, 23] Cream (tretinoin .02% or .05%) is approved by the FDA for treatment of *fine* wrinkles (such as those around the eyes), but it will not remove deep wrinkles. The cream must be used for many months before any reduction in the fine wrinkles will be noticed. If you use Renova, and skin irritation occurs, discontinue use or use it less frequently and apply an unscented moisturizer (such as Moisturel Lotion or Purpose Lotion) before applying Renova.

Other creams can make skin feel tight, with the sensation of wrinkle reduction, but that does not mean that the wrinkles are going away. If you've found a cream that you like, think that it is improving your appearance, and it doesn't irritate your skin, go ahead and use it. But don't pay an exorbitant amount of money for a "wrinkle-cure" cream. It's just not out there yet.

I've read that Botox can get rid of wrinkles, lift eyebrows, and take years off of a person's appearance. Is that true?

—*Scarlet, age 51*

Botulinum toxin injections (Botox)[24] can "relax" wrinkles by blocking nerves to locally paralyze muscles under the skin that affect wrinkles.

The toxin is produced by bacteria (Clostridium botulinum), which cause a type of food poisoning. The injections can be used to relax wrinkles between the eyebrows, at the corners of the eyes ("crows' feet"), and on the forehead. Where injected, the toxin "depletes" substances from nerve endings in the muscles. This causes muscles to relax, and wrinkles become smooth. The results last about three or four months.

Side effects can include temporary dry mouth and rarely, eyelid or brow drooping, flu-like symptoms, and muscle weakness. For effects to continue, the injections must be repeated every three or four months. Botox injections can also be used to decrease sweating of hands (palms), feet (soles), and underarms.

TREATMENT OF CELLULITE

What is cellulite? It is not a term used by all physicians since it is simply a "dressed up" term that means fat and lax skin. Fat cells in skin are normally contained within a number of partitioned compartments made of fibers ("fibrous septa"). As a person puts on weight, fat cells multiply and become larger, bulging against these septa and creating the lumpy, bumpy look of "cellulite." To make things worse, as a person ages, the skin becomes more lax. Fibrous septa remain, and "dimpling" of skin occurs, resulting in the picture of what is commonly called "cellulite."

How can you reduce cellulite? The simple truth is eat less, exercise more. What if that doesn't work? Is there anything else that can help? You can try liposuction, where fibrous septa are disrupted and fat cells are suctioned away. As described earlier in this chapter, there are risks involved in liposuction, but it can be effective in removing fat.

What about herbal creams and massage? Advertisements that promote herbal creams and massage claim that increasing vascular flow and lymphatic drainage will help reduce "cellulite." No cream or massage alone is going to get rid of the dimpled fat. Eat a well-balanced diet with reduced calories and fat, and exercise regularly!

CHAPTER 9

PROTECT YOUR CHILD'S SKIN

On the way home from the hospital with our little baby girl, I panicked. I mean—this is my first baby! How will I know what to do! Can I bathe her with soap? Or do I need some sort of special cleanser? Or special lotions? Please help!

—*Monica, age 25*

NEWBORN SKIN IS SPECIAL

There's nothing more precious than a baby. And Monica will do just fine. But there are some important things to know about baby skin.

Mild Soap and Moisturizer

Baby skin usually holds moisture well, but if the skin surface is damaged by harsh soaps or other substances, then infections and other problems can occur. Use non-perfumed soaps and if your baby has dry skin, apply an unscented moisturizer after bathing your baby.

Gentle Shampoo

A gentle shampoo that does not irritate eyes, such as Johnson's No More Tears, is very important. Avoid using your adult shampoo that can irritate eyes—some of the suds will inevitably get in baby's eyes.

Body Surface Area and Topical Applications

Because a baby has a relatively large body surface area in relation to its weight, lotions and other topical applications are absorbed in higher concentrations than in an adult. Be careful what you apply, and apply only as needed.

Sun Protection

Keep your baby out of the direct sun and dress him or her in protective clothing. The risks and benefits of using sunscreens on babies under six months old are not yet known, so keep baby out of direct sun. After your baby is six months old he or she should still stay out of the sun as much as possible, and sunscreen should be applied to sun exposed areas.

Remember that the risk of skin cancer increases with sun exposure.

> **PROTECTING THE FUTURE OF YOUR BABY'S SKIN**
>
> - Keep your baby out of the sun as much as possible and apply sunscreen to sun-exposed areas.
> - Teach your child to apply sunscreen before going into the sun and to wear a hat when in direct sunlight for any period of time.

Sun damage is cumulative and the sun exposure that a young child receives contributes to an increased risk of skin cancer in later life. In fact, early blistering sunburns are a major risk factor for developing melanoma in later life.

Most sun exposure occurs before the age of eighteen, so you can make a big difference in the lives of your children by protecting them from the sun. Clothing for infants is available with up to SPF 15 protection. Your dermatologist can give you information[1] on where to order sun protective clothing for you and your baby.

PART II

SORTING TRUTH FROM HYPE

CHAPTER 10

ADVERTISEMENTS OR TRUTHS?

P inocchio couldn't get away with telling an untruth because his nose grew long with each lie. Even an exaggeration caused Pinocchio's nose to extend to embarrassingly enormous proportions.

Unfortunately even if this worked in real life, there's no way to see the noses of the advertising media. We see only the beautiful illustrations and appealing messages that prompt us to rush out and buy the latest product to preserve youth and beauty.

I saw this ad for a new cream that is supposed to prevent wrinkles. I'm ready to do anything to try to keep my skin young. Everywhere I look in the magazines I see lotions and creams that are supposed to "turn back the clock" on aging. "How can I know what's really true?"

—Lucia, age 25

Books and magazine articles abound with new things to try. Advertisements make astounding claims about proprietary mixtures of herbs, perfumes, potions, teas, oils, and other natural substances. You'll find it all, presented with incredible imagery. You will see everything claimed for any given product.

What do consumers hope for? The single, miracle product that "does it all." The product that "reverses aging." The lotion that turns the consumer into a beautiful model. The new gadget that removes unwanted hair permanently and painlessly. The new miracle treatment for acne. The new product that smoothes out skin color, does away with uneven skin tones. The magic creams that melt way "cellulite."

Whatever the consumer wants, industries and the advertisers will promote. Remember, though, that advertisements are enticements, *not* news bulletins.

I bought this new gadget that was supposed to get rid of facial hairs. You just hold it up to the hairs, turn it on, and away go the hairs forever, or so the advertisement claimed. It cost a lot, but I thought it would be worth it if I didn't have to keep plucking those awful chin hairs. Well, it was a joke. A bad joke. When I got it I saw that it was just some new way to pluck hairs.

I called the company, but they wouldn't take it back. I threw it away. I got burned. But how can you know what really works and what doesn't

—Laurie, age 32

Stay with products from the well-known cosmetic and health care companies. They are more likely to have conducted adequate safety studies prior to introducing a new "gadget" or prior to including a "natural product" in a lotion or cosmetic. These companies also have a reputation to maintain, and "gadgets" that don't work well can tarnish that reputation. Nevertheless, even the best-known companies can stretch truth in advertising their products.

I saw this ad the other day for a new "all-in-one" cream that has the strength of prescription creams in getting down in skin to get rid of wrinkles. It's supposed to give the results of a face lift. The model in the ad didn't have a wrinkle or a sag anywhere on her face—she must have been in her 40's but she looked about 22. If something is this strong, won't it really do something for my skin?

—Danielle, age 35

If an ingredient is strong enough to cause a true drug-like result, then it will likely be a drug requiring prescription by a physician, with FDA-approval. FDA-approval means that the industry has proved to the FDA that the product works.

But over-the-counter products can be marketed without FDA approval. The product will be sold on "claims" that it works, but there's been no proof submitted to the FDA that it does work. Over-the-counter creams and lotions may smell good, moisturize and soothe skin. They may make skin feel soft and diminish the *appearance* of wrinkles, but they are not going to get down deep enough in skin to *cure* wrinkles and make skin regain its youthfulness. Not yet, anyway.

I just read about a new discovery that will get rid of wrinkles, and I can't wait to buy it! It must be true, because the advertisement says that it's based on a scientific discovery. Scientists found that algae living in "hot spots" way down on the ocean hold the secret to eternal youthfulness, and they are putting this discovery into a new oil to eliminate wrinkles!

—Madeline, age 35

Can we believe an advertisement because it says that a new product is based on scientific discovery? "Scientific discovery" and "scientists" are general terms. Where's the proof? What scientists? Advertisements can claim just about anything. And they will.

A new cream is being promoted in the popular magazines to answer our hopes and dreams. The model has beautiful, blemish-free skin. The cream is a breakthrough developed by a doctor. It is sold through the doctor's Web site. Can we believe the claims?

A new book has come out that says that the secrets of the ages have been unlocked and for the first time ever we now know how to turn back the clock and really look like we did when we were twenty! A number of new products have been developed based on these secrets, and are available now in the stores. In small print you notice that the author is president of a company that develops anti-aging products. Can we believe this book?

An Internet site gives information about health products and announces an essential oil that will melt away wrinkles. Looks like a reliable site. Comments on the site about the oil are by a physician. There is more information there about diabetes, Alzheimers, other medical problems. So the information must be true about the essential oil! You can order it with one click. It's not an educational site, but it is a physician's office, so shouldn't the information be reliable? Can we believe this?

We want to believe. More than anything. We'd love to melt away wrinkles and look like we did when we were twenty! We'd like to look like a beautiful model! But look carefully. The examples given are advertising in disguise.

How does advertising continue to draw so many consumers to products if the advertising is built on hype? Because the average consumer goes on to try another product before it is evident that the first doesn't work as claimed.

Let's say you see an advertisement for making your skin ten years younger. Sure wouldn't hurt to try, you decide. You try some of the products. So do your friends. They seem to work! Your skin is smoother, softer. The expensive prices are worth it! You are excited. Two months later you see another advertisement. This product is going to give you baby skin. Healthy, soft to the touch, beautiful! Sure wouldn't hurt to try! Why not give the new product a try, you decide.

And so on it goes. There's always a new spin, a new ingredient, a new promise, a new hope. There's usually no harm unless your skin becomes irritated, which sometimes happens, or your pocketbook suffers. But don't be led down the path of believing that new products that emerge are a *necessity* for good skin care. Good skin care, to repeat, requires a mild soap, a moisturizer if your face is dry, and a sunscreen. That's it, pure and simple.

The good news is that in the not-to-distant future we really will have new products that have remarkable effects. Industry and academia are collaborating more closely together than ever to translate basic research into products useful to healthcare and to the consumer. Billions of dollars are going into support of research that is leading to ideas that will be translated into exciting new cosmetics with real cosmeceutical effects and into new drugs and new medical therapies that will make a tremendous difference to society. Chapter 29 discusses what's ahead for us.

FIVE STEPS FOR SORTING TRUTH FROM ILLUSION

As we move into the future, the problem remains. How does one sort out what is true from what is "the sale of an illusion"? Here are five steps for doing just that.

First, determine if what you are reading is advertising in disguise. Advertising in a site that appears educational or otherwise objective, makes a claim appear real. Consider whether the author has self-interest in what is discussed. Will the person or organization mentioning a Web site, book, or article profit in any way from the sale of a product advertised there? Sometimes it's hard to tell. If a physician's office sells a product or owns a company that sells a product, the physician profits. If an organization gives medical information to promote a product, look at the nature of the organization. Is it an educational (.edu), governmental (.gov), or non-profit association unlikely to profit from sales of the product? Is it is a .com organization that will profit from sales?

Second, look to a reliable Web site for more information. Use search engines to locate information about a product on the Internet. Your search will turn up a mix of advertisements and useful sites. Go to the educational Web sites first. University and Medical School Web sites can give abundant information about health and treatments for disorders. Their Web addresses will usually contain ".edu." As mentioned above, aim for .edu or .gov Web sites or those that do not contain ".com." A long list of Web sites is available in the Appendix that will be helpful to you. You can find literature references to new compounds on PubMed.[1] Reputable magazines such as *Science*, or *Nature*, or *Scientific American* may contain articles, apart from advertisements, about a new type of product. Make sure you do not see the word, "advertisement," anywhere on the page.

Third, check with your physician. Good products are advertised just as are other products. The important thing to determine is whether the product will do what is claimed and whether it is right for you.

Fourth, stick with products from well-known cosmetic or pharmaceutical companies. Learn which industries have close collaboration with academic scientists to understand the likelihood that innovative new products will emerge from that industry. Look at the Web sites of the companies whose products you like. Are they interacting in a significant way to stay abreast of research findings? Are they collaborating with researchers? If so, their Web site should reflect this.

Five, remember the bottom line. A cream or lotion without irritating properties may be a good moisturizer. But it's not going to make your skin twenty years younger. The appearance of fine wrinkles can be minimized, but deep wrinkles will not be affected unless the dermis is treated with deep peels, with laser treatment, or with a face lift. Few creams can penetrate past the outer layer of the epidermis. Some hair growth can be stimulated by certain products, but we still cannot make bald heads regrow a full head of hair. Skin aging can be minimized by sun protection, but our skin still shows pigmentary changes, wrinkling, and sagging with time.

Six, remember the basics. You need a mild soap for cleansing your face, a moisturizer if your skin is dry, and a sunscreen. That's it. Pure and simple.

Build upon the basics within this book and seek truth from your own research and from your physician as new products arise. Continue to learn from the many sources available.

Finally, this chapter isn't designed to take away hope. It's to give a realistic picture of where we are today in skin care. The products on the marketplace serve important functions. Skin creams and lotions moisturize, protect the skin barrier, and improve appearance by offsetting skin dryness. Sunscreens protect against sun damage including skin aging caused by sun exposure. Bleaching creams can help lighten some types of dark patches on skin. Certain over-the-counter skin products can remove hair temporarily.

> **HOW TO SORT TRUTH FROM HYPE**
>
> • First, determine if what you are reading is advertising in disguise.
> • Second, look to a reliable Web site for more information.
> • Third, check with your physician.
> • Fourth, stick with products from well-known cosmetic or pharmaceutical companies.
> • Five, remember the bottom line: It won't cure wrinkles
> • Six, remember the basics.

You are the ultimate judge of a product. If you like it and think that it is helping your skin and you are not having any problems with your skin, use it! Just realize what it what it will and what it won't do. Be an educated consumer and seek the truth!

CHAPTER 11

GETTING PAST THE MYTHS
AND HANG-UPS

You may be surprised that you don't need a battery of skin care products such as alpha-hydroxy acids, antioxidants, and vitamin preparations. In fact, if your skin is irritated, one of these may be the culprit. What's the real story about these products? And what about spas and facials? Do they help?

ALPHA-HYDROXY ACIDS

I used to read a lot about how a good skin care regimen should include an alpha-hydroxy acid product to clean off dead skin and get rid of wrinkles. I haven't heard much about this recently, but I'm hearing about other creams that appear important. Are alpha-hydroxy acid products still an important part of a skin care regimen?

—Diane, age 37

Alpha-hydroxy acid (AHA) products are often promoted to make skin smooth and wrinkle-free. They can make your skin smooth, but there is no firm evidence that they significantly affect wrinkles.

What these products essentially do is remove the outer layer of dead skin. The mild acid irritates skin, and irritated skin stimulates skin repair, which results in newer skin. Mild facial peels (e.g., glycolic acid peels) as well as some face creams often contain alpha-hydroxy acid.

AHA products can be helpful in smoothing sun-damaged skin, in helping reduce some dark spots on skin from sun-damage, and in treating acne. AHA products are sometimes used with bleaching agents to increase the efficiency of the bleaching agents.

On the "down" side, they can produce mild skin irritation that can sometimes disrupt your protective skin barrier. They can also increase the risk of sunburn.

The bottom line is that it is not necessary to incorporate AHAs into your daily routine. You may do so if you like, but there is no long-term benefit to your skin in their use. There is no need to irritate your skin every day, even slightly. If you use an AHA product, be sure to wear a sunscreen and discontinue using the product if your skin becomes irritated.

VITAMIN PREPARATIONS

I don't have wrinkles now, thank goodness, but what should I be doing now to prevent wrinkles in the future? I'm only 22, but I know that wrinkles are lurking down the road. I've heard that Renova will prevent wrinkles. Should I be using it every day? Will it—or something else—really prevent wrinkles?
—Bonnie, age 38

Renova is derived from tretinoin, the acid form of Vitamin A. Other tretinoin products include Retin-A and Avita. Tretinoin products are useful for treatment of fine wrinkles and for treatment of acne.

Although tretinoin won't *prevent* wrinkling, it can *treat* fine wrinkles. Renova is currently the only FDA-approved cream for treatment of fine wrinkles.

Remember that the most common cause of premature wrinkling is sun exposure. The best prevention of wrinkles, therefore, is protection from the sun by use of sunscreen and protective clothing.

Unless prescribed by your dermatologist, there is no need to routinely apply tretinoin, or any other vitamin preparation. Use a mild soap, moisturizer, and sunscreen as your basic skin care regimen.

I've heard that Vitamin E helps wounds heal and prevents scars. Is this true?
—Bobby, age 32

There is no conclusive data to show that Vitamin E is helpful in wound healing or treatment of scars. Vitamin E can irritate skin, just as can other vitamin preparations. Get your vitamins through a well-balanced diet. They'll go where they are supposed to—they'll get to the skin from the "inside out" in the appropriate amount that nature intended.

ANTIOXIDANTS

But aren't the antioxidant properties of vitamin E and other vitamins important to skin?
—Carol, age 38

Yes, Vitamin E and Vitamin C, as well as other substances in skin are antioxidants important to healthy skin. During metabolism our body constantly generates "free radicals." Larger amounts of free radicals are generated during cellular injury, such as when UV irradiation of skin occurs. These free radicals are unstable molecules that oxidize and destroy other molecules. Cellular damage by free radicals plays a role in the aging process and in many diseases.

Damaged cells that cannot be repaired normally die[1] and are cleaned up by cells called macrophages that move around and engulf the dead cells. Some cell death is necessary for a healthy body. Old cells and cells that are damaged and cannot be repaired are supposed to die. Mopping up *all* free radicals is not necessarily the best thing. It is the right balance that is important.

Your skin contains antioxidants that "mop up" excess free radicals, blocking the destructive process ("oxidative stress") that results from an overabundance of free radicals. When oxidative stress occurs, it is too much for the macrophages to handle—too many dead cells to clean up. By the time the macrophages get around to cleaning up all of the debris, the residual debris and damaged cells have not only "clogged up the works," but they may also have triggered damaging immune responses. Some of the cells with damaged DNA may have multiplied.

Supplying more antioxidants to the skin would seem to be the answer to preventing damage from excessive free radicals, and a well-balanced diet rich in fruits and vegetables will help you maintain appropriate antioxidants. But will antioxidants work topically?

There are two obstacles to overcome: (1) Putting an antioxidant on the skin does not necessarily result in getting it inside the skin and inside the cells, where it needs to be. The benefits of vitamin E as a protective skin antioxidant occur inside the skin and inside the cells, not on the skin surface. (2) Even if the antioxidant does get into the skin, what effect is it going to have there? It's the *balance* of substances inside the cell that's important. Nature has carefully fine-tuned the cell's interactions. Even with the right intentions, it's hard to reach the desired effect without throwing something else off balance. There are also other factors to consider. Under UVB exposure, for example, vitamin E may actually *induce* oxidative stress and act as a photosensitizer, interfering with the normal cytokine signals, and oxidizing important targets in cells and biological fluids.

Scientists are vigorously studying antioxidants and their effects.[2] Cosmetic companies are eager to incorporate new findings into their product strategies. The future should hold many exciting applications of this research. In the meantime, keep eating fruits and vegetables. They are high in vitamins, minerals, flavonoids, and carotenoids, that have been shown to have high antioxidant properties and will give your body the tools that it needs to fine-tune and balance its antioxidative functions.

SPAS, AROMATHERAPY, FACIALS—WILL THEY HELP?

My one indulgence is a weekly facial. When I'm having the facial, I'm in another world. I feel so relaxed, and during the day when I'm in a stressful meeting, I can think about my facials and feel myself relax. They are wonderful! But recently my face has been breaking out with acne—and I'm way past my acne years!

—Andrea, age 47

Spas, Aromatherapy, and Facials are designed to soothe, relax, diminish stress. A massage with quiet, slow music and fragrant scent to the air can transport you away from your daily problems to an oasis of relaxation and pleasure. So yes, they help—they help you relax. Stress can affect skin and body condition in many ways. It's always good to eliminate stress.

A word of caution—fragrant soaps and lotions can cause skin irritation. Vigorous massage of the face can stimulate sebaceous glands and cause acne. If your face or other parts of your skin begin to break out while indulging in these activities, back off a little and use other stress-reducing activities, such as exercise.

CHAPTER 12

ALTERNATIVE THERAPIES, NATURAL PRODUCTS, FACT OR FICTION?

A re "natural products" best? What about herbs, tea extracts, hydroxyacids, essential oils, and fatty acids? Is there any benefit in using these substances, or is what you hear just advertising hype?"

HERBS, VITAMINS, AND "NATURAL" PRODUCTS

I use only natural products on my skin. I take herbal supplements as well as shark's fin, hemlock essence, marigold bud, and oil of hedgehog. I want to do the best for my body and skin. But lately I've been itching all over and have this red rash everywhere!

—Julie, age 51

In ancient days, medical therapeutics consisted mostly of herbal therapies and other potions. A medicine man, or witch doctor, or whoever administered to the sick would learn from those who came before him what might work and what would not. There was an aura of mystery around such "medicine men," who would magically heal the sick with special potions. There were no pharmaceutical products at the drug store—everything had to be made from "natural" products in the world around them.

Today many of the old remedies have been incorporated into effective over-the-counter products and into prescription medicines found in drug stores. Many new uses of "natural substances" have been discovered. For example, Aloe vera, a component of many soothing lotions, comes from herbs. Digoxin, the cardiac medication, comes from the foxglove plant. There are many other examples of current day therapies derived from natural products; see Table 12.1.

These are only some of the current day medical therapies derived from natural products, and there are continuing efforts by the federal government to detect new and useful therapies from natural substances and other sources.[1]

There is indeed a certain comfort in knowing that an ingredient is found in nature and is not "man-made." The term, "natural ingredients," sounds as though the product should be good for you, and so advertising campaigns are

Table 12.1. Current Treatments Derived from Natural Products

Product	Source	Use
Aloe vera	from herbs	Soothing lotions
Penicillins and cephalosporins (Keflex, others)	from bread mold	Antibiotic
Vinca alkaloids	from periwinkle plant	Used by oncologists to treat cancer
Psoralen (furocoumarin)	from food plants (eg. parsnip, celery, limes)	Used to treat psoriasis and other diseases (PUVA treatment: psoralen +UVA)
Podophyllin	from the root of the American mayapple	Applied to treat genital or perianal Warts
Tannic acid	from seaweed	Used to treat burns

quick to jump to this opportunity to blend what appears true and appealing with advertising hype.

Remember that "natural" is a very broad term meaning anything found "in nature." Many "natural" products are not meant to be ingested or applied to the skin.

The needles of the hemlock tree are "natural," but they can kill you if you eat them. Likewise the bark of the beautiful oleander tree can kill you if you eat it. Poison ivy is a "natural product" that you don't want to rub on your skin.

The bottom line is that there can be allergens, irritants, and poisons in "natural" ingredients that can be bad for you. The phrase, "natural product" doesn't automatically equate to "good for you."

> *I know that everything found is nature may not be good for the body, but someone selling a product isn't going to want to sell something that would make me sick or irritate my skin. I feel comfortable that anything that my health food store sells is going to be safe.*
>
> *—Roxanne, age 32*

In deciding whether to try a "natural" product from a health food store, the questions are:

Does it work?
Is it safe?

Before a *drug* can go into the marketplace, the U.S. Federal Drug Administration (FDA) must decide that the drug (1) works as claimed, and (2) is safe. Proving to the FDA that a drug works and is safe is an arduous process for the drug manufacturer.

After the preliminary studies in the scientific laboratory, the drug must be tested in animals, and then if it appears safe and effective in animals, the manufacturer applies to the FDA for permission to try the drug in humans. After all of the tests are completed, the results are presented to the FDA for careful review and consideration of all of the data to decide whether the drug can be released for production and sale. By the time a drug reaches the drugstore for a physician to prescribe, it has been through numerous controlled tests and has been found safe and effective in both animals and in humans.

This is not so with herbal and other "natural" products. The FDA does not usually evaluate over-the-counter supplements, and therefore there is no guarantee of product quality, safety, or efficacy.

I know that herbs and other natural products are not approved by the government, but the advertisements say that lots of tests have been done to show that the products work. I even looked on the Internet and found reports of studies in some of the scientific publications.

—*Stewart, age 41*

There are many variables that influence the outcome of a study and many ways that a study can be presented. If you look hard enough, you can find respectable references for whatever you want to find. Don't like spinach, though you know it's good for you, and want to feel OK about not eating it? The Cambridge World History of Foods[2] points out that spinach contains oxalic acid that builds kidney stones and interferes with the body's absorption of calcium. Don't like lima beans? They are a great source of iron, protein, and fiber. But do you want to find a reference that says they are not good for you? You are in luck. The same source[3] points out that lima beans contain cyanide. Take it all, but not literally, with a grain of salt. That goes for the benefits of herbal remedies, too.

There are hundreds of anecdotal claims that one herb or another is

NECESSARY STUDIES

- Studies should be conducted in *non-biased settings*, such as in a university or medical center—not within the industry producing the product.
- There should be controls where those not using the product are compared with those using the product.
- The studies should be "blinded"—that is, no one should know which group is using the product and which are using the controls until after the entire test period is over.
- There should be human clinical trials (studies in humans) as well as animal studies. Good outcomes in animals does not automatically mean good outcomes in humans.

effective for a particular medical problem. Often there are no controlled studies to prove it. But even if there are studies—even if the studies are reported in the scientific literature—they must be interpreted with caution.

Remember that whether a herb or "natural" substance works or not is only half of the equation. The question remains as to whether or not it is safe. Even if it is safe for the problem treated, there may be side effects under certain conditions that are not beneficial. Herb therapy, ingested or applied topically, can affect other medications. Some oral therapies should not be used by pregnant or nursing women.

Table 12.2. Claims and Side Effects of Herbs and "Natural" Substances

Substance	Advertised Claims	Side Effects
Ginkgo biloba	Improve memory and concentration	Increased bleeding during surgical procedures
Feverfew	Reduce fever, migraines, and arthritic complaints	Increased bleeding during surgical procedures
Garlic	Lower cholesterol and promote healthy heart	Increased bleeding during surgical procedures
Ginger	Increase digestion	Increased bleeding during surgical procedures
Asian ginseng	Sexual health	Increased bleeding during surgical procedures; elevate blood pressure
Vitamin E, oral	antioxidant	Increased bleeding during surgical procedures
Vitamin E, topical	Wound healing, reduce scarring	Skin irritation
Ephedra	Promote weight loss	Can interact with epinephrine (usually included in topical anesthetics prior to skin surgery or dental work) to cause cardiac stress
St. John's Wort	Help maintain emotional balance and positive outlook	Increases risk of sunburn; can interact with many medicines, including the heart medicine, digoxin; can interact with cyclosporine (used by organ transplant patients), increasing the risk of organ transplant rejection.
Tee Tree Oil	Applied for moisturizing, healing skin	Can cause skin irritation (allergic contact dermatitis)

Some herbs increase the risk of bleeding during surgical procedures. Others can stress your heart. Some make your skin more likely to sunburn.

It is important to tell your physician about any "natural products" that you are using. More information is needed about alternative medicines to determine effectiveness and safety. Table 12.2 provides just a few examples of problems that can occur.

What if you are convinced that your favorite herbal product does work for you. You've never looked so good. You know that it helps your skin. It is not causing any problems. Then if it works for you, use it. But remember that there can be potential side effects. If irritation or rash develops, stop using the product immediately and revert to the tried and true, basic beauty routine: mild soap, moisturizer, and sunscreen. If the problem does not resolve, see your dermatologist. You can cause harm by jumping from one herbal product to another trying to treat a problem by yourself.

The best advice is to keep your beauty routine basic and simple, get sufficient rest and eat a balanced diet. Your skin will glow with health from simple, good care.

See the Appendix for reports of benefits from other alternative therapies.

CHAPTER 13

NEW "BREAKTHROUGH PRODUCTS": DO THEY WORK?

The FDA has acknowledged in the past that "Most cosmetics contain ingredients that are promoted with exaggerated claims of beauty or long-lasting effects to create an image.[1] Image is what the cosmetic industry sells through its products, and it's up to the consumer to believe it or not."

But consumers are becoming frustrated with the exaggerated claims, or "puffery," and are becoming more and more unwilling to spend hard-earned money on products that will not work as advertised. They are excited that scientists continue to search for breakthroughs, but they are looking for more realistic claims of the products that they buy.

But where are we now? Let's look at some of the new products on the marketplace and see what they do, and what they don't do.

New moisturizers are in development that help keep the skin from cracking and drying after showering. Olay Ribbons Body Wash, for example, is a product designed to combine cleansing agents with moisturizing agents to prevent skin dryness. While this is not a novel idea (Many soaps such as Dove soap contain "moisturizing ingredients"), the new product does make skin feel silky and soft.

New "home products" to stimulate skin and help remove dead cells are in development. The Clarisonic Skin Care Brush, developed by the inventor of the Sonicare Toothbrush, has been developed to "deeply cleanse, stimulate, and clarify" skin. Although gentle cleansing with your hands is sufficient to cleanse skin, the Skin Care Brush will serve to remove dead skin in a manner similar to microdermabrasion. Be careful not to overuse, and stop using if there is excessive irritation. Remember that overly-aggressive cleaning can cause acne to flare.

Among the myriad of "antiwrinkle" creams are products containing Retinol or other ingredients claimed to have some effect upon fine wrinkles, but they likely work most effectively as moisturizers to smooth skin. The only FDA-approved treatment for fine wrinkles is the prescription product, Renova. That's not to say that "antiwrinkle" creams won't help skin look better. Any good moisturizer, however, will help keep moisture in the outer layer of skin, giving the appearance of smoother skin.

New over-the-counter creams that contain a group of amino acids called "pentapeptides" are also among the creams claimed to remove wrinkling. It is doubtful that any active ingredients would penetrate deep enough to remove wrinkles, and as other antiwrinkle creams, the primary benefit is likely in moisturizing the skin.

Copper peptides have been added to many skin care products with the claim that they support and improve skin healing and prevent skin aging. References to animal and human tests appear to support enhancement of wound healing. Support of anti-aging however, appears more tangential.

Strivectin is promoted as a wrinkle-reducing cream containing an oligo-peptide called Pal-KTTKS. The manufacturer, Klein-Becker, does not offer any explanation as to how it claims that the product works, only that it was a "remarkable turn of events" that some people using the cream to try to treat stretch marks used it on the face and had favorable results. It is very unlikely that a large molecule such as an oligo-peptide could penetrate past the upper layer of skin. As with other creams and lotions, the primary effect of this product is likely a moisturizing one.

Argeriline is the trademark name of a synthetic molecule acetyl hexapeptide-3, claimed by its promoters to relax facial muscles and thereby reduce wrinkles in the same way as BOTOX® injections. It is doubtful that this molecule penetrates the skin deeply enough in its commercial concentration to create such effect. Moreover, Botox must be injected into certain muscles to give the desired effect of lifting face and brow and decreasing wrinkles. Certain other facial muscles are not injected, to reduce the chance of facial sagging. If any cream rubbed over the face did actually penetrate muscles, it would likely do so non-selectively, resulting in facial sagging.

Heliocare[2] is an oral dietary supplement with antioxidant properties which helps maintain the skin's ability to protect against sun related effects. Protection against sun damage helps prevent photoaging. Other supplements are also in development that may give added protection against sun damage, both before and after sun exposure. Look for this area of photoprotection to expand in the near future. Remember, however, do not rely on oral supplements alone. The experience with such supplements in still in the early stages, and it is of vital importance to protect from sun in other ways, including application of sunscreens that protect against both UVB and UVA radiation.

It is important to remember that there are many, many peptides within skin that facilitate wound healing, protect skin against sun exposure, enhance cell turnover, eliminate substances within skin that contribute to the effects of aging, stimulate substances in skin that contribute to skin firmness and elasticity, and participate in other skin functions.

The breakthrough cream in the future will be a balance of important signals in skin contained in a vehicle that will penetrate to appropriate skin depths to create the desired effect. Nanotechnology, discussed in Chapter 36, provides the tools to accomplish such penetration. Already products are in the market-place using this technology. But we are just on the threshold of utilizing the "nanoworld" for therapeutic purposes. Only time will tell how effectively and safely it will be utilized. Our hats go off to those who diligently search for impor-tant signals within skin, but it is important to limit claims to those that can be reasonably expected from the data presented.

PART III

A SKIN CARE PROGRAM FOR YOUR SKIN

CHAPTER 14

THE HEALTHY SKIN PROGRAM

W e all want beautiful skin, renewed confidence, a new outlook on life. We all want our skin look ten years younger, heads to turn in admiration.

So let's get started! The Healthy Skin Program is not about new astringents, apricot balms, eye emollients, or scrubs. It's about healthy, attractive skin that reflects a healthy body.

First, let's assess your skin. Get a pencil and circle your answers to the following questions. Add any of your own comments or clarifications beside your answers.

1. SKIN TYPE

What best fits your skin type? These are the Fitzpatrick skin types. In 1975, Fitzpatrick,[1] a dermatologist, created this standard for classifying individuals according to their skin type.

Type I: Always burn, never tan, very white skin, freckles, blonde or red hair, blue or green eyes.

Type II: Usually burn, sometimes tan, have white skin, blond hair, blue or green eyes.

Type III: Sometimes burn, usually tan, white to olive skin, brown hair, and brown eyes.

Type IV: Rarely burn, always tan, brown skin, brown or black hair, brown eyes.

Type V: Very rarely burn, dark brown skin, dark brown to black hair.

Type VI: Never burn, dark skin, black hair.

The lower the skin type number, the greater the risk of skin cancer from sun exposure. If you are Type I or II, sun protection is vital to reduce the risk of sunburn. Use at least SPF 30 and wear sun-protective clothing such as hats and sunglasses. Even though burning may not occur often in types III—VI, damage to skin cells can nevertheless occur, so sun protection is still important. Use SPF 15 or greater.

2. SKIN OILINESS

Is your skin:

(1) Dry
(2) Oily in the "T" Zone (nose and forehead above eyes); dry outside the "T" Zone
(3) Oily

If your skin is dry, a mild unscented soap such as Dove or Cetaphil soap is important. Pat dry and apply a small amount of unscented moisturizer such as Moisturel Lotion or Purpose Lotion.

If your skin is oily, use a soap such as Purpose Soap or Neutrogena soap. A salicylic acid wash (Neutrogena and other skin care companies make these) can also be useful in removing excess oil from skin. Rinse well, and pat dry. Do not apply moisturizer unless your skin becomes dry.

If your skin has "combination" dryness and oiliness—such as oily in the "T" zone and dry outside the "T" zone, use a mild soap such as Dove. This can be followed by a salicylic acid wash over oily areas and Moisturel Lotion or Purpose Lotion sparingly in the dry areas.

3. MOOD

What's your mood?

(1) Happy almost all of the time
(2) Happy most of the time
(3) Moody
(4) Depressed
(5) Stressed

If you are depressed, see a psychologist or psychiatrist for treatment. Take action now to address any underlying problems. Fill your mind with optimism and happy thoughts. Your appearance will reflect good care of body, mind, and spirit. If you are often stressed, include stress-reducing exercises in your daily routine.

4. SUNSCREEN

Do you wear sunscreen?

(1) Always
(2) Sometimes
(3) Never

Always wear a sunscreen to prevent photoaging and to reduce the risk of skin cancer.

5. PERFUMED PRODUCTS

Do you wear perfumed lotions or use perfumed soaps?

(1) Never
(2) Sometimes
(3) Always

If you have any skin problems, avoid perfumed lotions or perfumed soaps. Perfume is a skin irritant. Dab a little perfume on your clothing if you want to wear it, but keep it away from your skin.

6. HEALTH

Are you in good health?

(1) Yes
(2) Some health problems
(3) No

Address any health problems. Your skin reflects your health.

7. EXERCISE

Do you exercise?

(1) Never
(2) Sometimes
(3) Regularly

Have an exercise program and stick to it. You'll be healthier and happier and your skin will reflect this.

8. WEIGHT

Are you

(1) Overweight?
(2) The ideal weight?
(3) Underweight?

If you are overweight or underweight, see your physician to develop a sensible diet and STICK TO IT. Take action NOW.

9. APPETITE

Is your appetite

(1) Too good?
(2) Normal?
(3) Bad?

If your appetite is too good, exercise more, take yourself away from the refrigerator. Get out of the house if necessary to get away from food. If your appetite is bad and you are feeling bad, see your physician for a checkup.

10. HAPPINESS

Are you happy?

(1) Most of the time
(2) Sometimes
(3) Occasionally

Your skin reflects your attitude. If there are situations that keep you unhappy, see a counselor—psychologist or psychiatrist—to talk about the problems and develop a plan to address the situations. Don't put this off. Correct what you can, work towards problems, find things that make you happy, and put yourself in an environment so that you can be happy. When you are taking all the action that you can—doing what you can—then focus on the positive. Action—correction—optimism—positivity—happiness.

11. SLEEP

How much sleep do you get each night on average?

(1) Seven hours or greater
(2) Five to seven hours
(3) Less than five hours

Most people need seven or eight hours of sleep per night. Go to bed. Unless you are on call as a doctor or for another profession, turn the phone off. Go to sleep.

12. RELAXATION

Do you take time to relax each day?

(1) No
(2) Sometimes
(3) Yes

Always take time to relax—even if it's for a minute several times a day. Stop—take a deep breath—exhale slowly. Close your eyes. Breathe slowly. You are on an island. No stress. No one around you. A gentle breeze—warm sunlight. Nothing else matters—for that minute.

Now, look back over your answers, and jot down any action on the Action Items page at the end of this chapter any action items from what you have circled thus far. For example, if your appetite is too good, list as action items (1) exercise more, and (2) take yourself away from the refrigerator. At the end of this chapter you'll turn the action item list into a Plan.

Next let's evaluate your complexion. Again, circle your answers.

13. COMPLEXION

Is your complexion:

(1) Clear?
(2) Blemished with acne?
(3) Itchy with rash?
(4) Sallow and colorless?
(5) Ruddy on cheeks and nose?
(6) With patchy darks spots?
(7) Wrinkled with sun damage?

(1) If clear, protect it with mild soap, moisturizer if skin is dry, and sunscreen. These are the Basics of Skin Care. Review Chapter 2 for more information.

(2) If blemished with acne, see your dermatologist for treatment.

- If there are painful cysts that leave scars, your dermatologist may prescribe an antibiotic as part of the treatment.
- In severe cases, isotretinoin may be prescribed.
- Try a salicylic wash (Neutrogena SalAc) or Purpose Soap for washing your face.
- You can try an over-the-counter benzoyl peroxide cream or gel (eg. Persagel) applied twice a day to the areas affected by acne, but if the acne does not resolve, see your dermatologist for treatment.

- Don't pick or squeeze pimples or cysts, or scarring can result.
- In cases of persistent whiteheads, your dermatologist may perform "acne surgery," or removal of the whiteheads one-by-one with a sterile instrument.
- In cystic acne, facial peels or intense pulsed light treatments may be helpful.
- See Chapter 18 for more information about acne.

(3) If itchy with rash, you may be allergic to a product that you are using on your face or to a medicine that you are taking or food that you are eating.

- Discontinue all facial products except a mild unscented soap such as Cetaphil and an unscented moisturizer such as Moisturel Lotion.
- See your dermatologist for treatment that will likely involve a very mild cortisone to apply twice a day until the rash resolves. Only the mildest cortisones should be applied to the face—medium strength or strong cortisone creams should never be used on the face.
- Your dermatologist may also prescribe an antihistamine to take for itching. Antihistamines can be taken by mouth for itching, but an antihistamine cream should never be applied to skin.
- Rashes can be caused by many different things. See your dermatologist for diagnosis and treatment.
- See Chapter 22 for more information about rash.

(4) If sallow and colorless, start an exercise program and eat a balanced diet.

- Get plenty of rest. The old adage, "Early to bed, early to rise makes a man (or woman) healthy, wealthy, and wise" still holds true.
- A little blush on the cheeks can help, but a natural blush from fresh air and exercise is much more attractive. Set aside a time to exercise *every single day!* Develop an exercise program that makes sense and stick to it.
- See your primary care physician for a check-up to make sure that any and all underlying health problems are addressed.
- Plan your diet rather than let your appetite lead you. Consult with a nutritionist or read a book on nutrition—not a diet book—to understand what proteins and minerals are necessary for a healthy body and what foods contain them. Balance your diet with an appropriate combination of lean meat, vegetables, whole grains, and fruit.
- See Chapter 5 for more information about healthy body-healthy skin.

(5) If ruddy on cheeks and nose, you may have rosacea. See your dermatologist for diagnosis.

- If you have rosacea, your dermatologist may prescribe a cream or gel such as Metrogel or Finacea.
- In severe cases, an antibiotic may be prescribed.
- Avoid things that make your face flush, such as wine, caffeine, spicy foods, hot temperatures.
- Be sure to wear a sunscreen. Sunlight causes rosacea to flare.
- Prominent blood vessels around the nose and on the cheeks can be treated cosmetically.

(6) If your skin has patchy darks spots, you need to protect your skin from the sun.

- See your dermatologist to make sure that these are benign "lentigines" ("sun:" or "age spots") and not a skin cancer or precancer.
- Sun protection is vital. Wear an SPF 45 or greater to protect from sun.
- Certain creams may be prescribed by your dermatologist to help fade these spots.
- Chemical peels can also help fade these spots.
- See Chapter 21 for more information about lentigines.

(7) If your skin is wrinkled with sun damage, you need to protect your skin from the sun and have a full skin exam every six months since you are at greater risk for developing skin cancer.

14. SUN DAMAGE

Next, let's assess the extent[2] of sun damage to your skin.

(1) Mild—Little wrinkles, no precancers
(2) Moderate—Early wrinkling, sallow complexion with early precancers
(3) Advanced—Persistent wrinkling, discoloration of the skin with telangiectasias and precancers
(4) Severe—Severe wrinkling, photoaging, gravitational and dynamic forces affecting skin, precancers with or without cancer

For **Mild** sun damage, you may need facial peels to even skin tone and renew skin surface. You will need regular skin checkups for detection and treatment of precancers or skin cancers. Always wear sunscreen. Avoid foundation makeup—adult acne may develop during these years, and foundation makeup will cause acne to flare.

For **Moderate** sun damage, Botox can be helpful to relax crows' feet and wrinkles between the eyebrows and on the forehead. Have regular checkups for detection and treatment of precancers or skin cancers, and wear sunscreen at all times.

For **Advanced** sun damage, Restylane injections can help fill in deep wrinkles above lips and between nose and mouth. Intense pulsed light or Fraxel treatments can help firm up skin and give a more youthful appearance. Botox can be used to treat crows' feet, forehead wrinkles, and wrinkles between the eyebrows. Laser or intense pulsed light can remove telangectasias (tiny blood vessels) on the face. CosmoPlast can restore an outline to lips. Have regular checkups for detection and treatment of precancers or skin cancers, and wear sunscreen at all times.

Use a little blush and eye makeup and some loose powder if you feel you must wear something on your skin, but avoid foundation makeup—it will clog pores and make you look older.

For **Severe** sun damage, appearance can be improved by the cosmetic procedures described for Advanced sun damage. In addition, you may also want to consider blepharoplasty to remove the droop from eyelids or a face lift to tighten and lift skin. Neck skin can also be "lifted." You may also be growing many "unwanted spots" (benign growths called "seborrheic keratoses") on your back and abdomen. Have these checked by your dermatologist to make certain of the diagnosis and to remove those that are itchy, otherwise irritated, or cosmetically objectionable (insurance does not usually cover removal for cosmetic purposes). Have regular checkups for detection and treatment of precancers or skin cancers, and wear sunscreen at all times.

Use a little blush and eye makeup and some loose powder if you feel you must wear something on your skin, but avoid foundation makeup—it will clog pores and wrinkles and make you look much, much older.

15. SKIN AGING

Do you have

(1) Deep lines from the nose to the corners of the mouth?
(2) A sagging neck?
(3) Old-looking hands?

- Restylane injections can soften deep lines from nose to mouth.
- See a plastic surgeon for treatment of a sagging neck.
- Injectible fillers such as collagen and elastin can help give a youthful appearance to old-looking hands. Bleaching agents and cryotherapy can erase some of the dark age spots on hands.

16. BAD HABITS

Do you have bad habits that affect your skin?

(1) Picking at acne spots
(2) Wearing lots of foundation makeup
(3) Trying new products all the time
(4) Frowning
(5) Not removing makeup before going to bed
(6) Not using soap to wash your face—you need soap to cleanse your face
(7) Not wearing sunscreen
(8) Putting too many things on your face

If you are doing any of these things, stop. Don't pick at acne spots—you'll cause scars and more acne will erupt around the picked spot. Don't wear foundation makeup. It clogs pores and can cause acne to erupt. Trying new products all the time is not bad, but you risk irritating your skin. If irritation occurs, go back to the basics. Don't frown—you *will* cause wrinkles. Be sure to remove makeup before going to bed. Otherwise you risk an acne flare-up. Use a mild, unscented soap to cleanse your face. Don't forget your sunscreen. Without it you are a setup for photoaging and at risk for developing skin cancer. There's no need to use a lot of products on your face. A mild soap for cleansing, a moisturizer if your face is dry, and a sunscreen. That's all you need for good skin care.

17. GOALS

What Are Your Goals for Your Appearance?

How do you want to look?
(1) Your age but not more
(2) Ten years younger
(3) A movie star
(4) A healthy, happy person

You can achieve and maintain healthy skin or completely change your appearance depending upon the goals that you set. Sit down before a mirror and decide what your goals will be. You can bring out the best in your skin as it is or you can literally shoot for the stars. Be bold!

(1) If you are happy looking your age with healthy skin, follow the guidelines for good skin care—stick to the basics. You can build upon the basics of skin care with a little makeup as suitable for you—lipstick, loose powder, blush, mascara—but keep the look natural. Exercise regularly to have a healthy glow to skin.

(2) If you want to look ten years younger, consider facial peels, facial resurfacing, intense pulsed light treatments, microdermabrasion, Fraxel
treatments, Sculptra or Restylane injections. See Chapter 8 for more
information about these treatments. See a plastic surgeon for other
options including face lifts.

(3) If you want to look like a movie star, see your plastic surgeon for
options. There are ways to augment chins and cheeks, revise noses,
augment breasts, and perform many other miracles for you.

(4) If you want to be a healthy, happy person, follow the guidelines in this
book for good skin care, see your primary care physician for a check-
up, exercise, eat a balanced diet, and take time for yourself to relax
and to have fun.

A DAILY PLAN

Now that you understand your skin type and its problems to remedy, set an
action plan according to your goals. Include:

- Daily skin care plan
- Subtle makeup to enhance, not cover
- Balanced diet
- Exercise plan
- Stress-reducing exercises
- Recreation
- Adequate sleep
- Relaxation and reflection

Sure, you say. If I didn't have to work full time, there might be time for
SOME of these items on the list—but there's no way to address all items . . .

Of course there is time. It's a matter of having a plan and sticking to it. How
to work it all in? Simple. Get a pencil and paper and make your PLAN.

Next go to your Action Plan and write down any additional information
necessary for carrying out your plan. If one of your items calls for seeing a dermatologist, look up the number of a dermatologist and write it down along with
the date that you will call for an appointment. If you do not have a dermatologist, write down how you will obtain recommendations (ask your primary care
physician, ask a friend) and write down the date for doing this. If another item
calls for taking stress breaks, set down the time and days (daily) that you will
have these breaks and how long you will allow for them. Continue making your
Plan in this manner, listing as much information as you can so that you won't
have to go to the phone book for numbers, won't have to make decisions later.

Avoid phrases in your Plan such as "as much as possible." Be definite. Be rea-
sonable. Be realistic. Be optimistic. If you think that you can't afford more than

2 minutes for a stress break, write down 2 minutes. You can always change the Plan as necessary, but start with a daily plan that addresses each item.

You will have added some of your own comments during the questionnaire. Address these comments in your plan.

Next, carry out your Plan. Don't procrastinate. Start now. Most of all, be excited about what you are about to do! You are going to look and feel fantastic!

Let's look at some sample plans.

A Plan for Jennifer

I'm the mother of two small children under three years old. I feel like I've really let myself go during the past three years, but there's just not time to do anything with these little ones keeping me so busy. How can I possibly make a Plan. I can't even take time out to think!

—Jennifer, age 24

1. **Skin Type**: Type II; **Action Plan**: At high risk for skin cancer; Use at least SPF 30 (daily) and wear sun-protective clothing such as hats and sunglasses (when in sun).
2. **Skin oiliness**: "T" Zone (nose and forehead above eyes) and dry outside the "T" Zone; **Action Plan**: Tomorrow buy Dove For Sensitive Skin and use for washing face. Buy Sal Ac Wash and use to wash over oily areas. Buy Moisturel Lotion for use in dry areas.
3. **Mood**: Happy most of the time, except often stressed.; **Action Plan**: include stress-reducing exercises in daily routine.
4. **Sunscreen**: Wear sunscreen sometimes.**Action Plan**: Buy sunscreen SPF 30 and wear daily.
5. **Perfumed products**: Wear sometimes. **Action Plan**: Avoid putting on skin. Can dab on clothing.
6. **Health**: In good health, just tired often. **Action Plan**: Factor in 15 minute nap when kids are taking nap. Plan to go to bed by 9 pm. Kids in bed by 8 pm.
7. **Exercise**: Sometimes. No time with kids keeping me busy. **Action Plan**: Buy exercise tape. 15 minutes in the living room each morning after children fed and while they are best at playing with toys.
8. **Weight**: OK. No time to eat. **Action Plan**: Balanced diet
9. **Appetite**: Normal, but tempted to snack; **Action Plan**: Eat small portions of healthy food, no snacking
10. **Happiness**: Most of the time. Sometimes feel overwhelmed. Love my kids but no time for myself. **Action Plan**: Discuss with Mark (husband) sharing responsibilities with the children before he goes to work or after he is home. Plan for babysitter at least once a week to go out to dinner with Mark or with friends.

11. **Sleep**: Five to seven hours. The baby wakes up at 6 am—if I'm lucky. Sometimes she is up at 2 pm for an hour. I'm exhausted in the morning. Can't go to bed early—that's the only time to clean the house, but I end up too exhausted for that at the end of the day. **Action Plan**: To bed by 9 pm every night. Arrange for help with cleaning.

12. **Relaxation**: No time to relax. Too much to do. Cleaning up behind the kids. Never have time to do any real house cleaning. **Action Plan**: Plan for help with cleaning. One minute relaxation break prior to 15 minute nap when kids put down for nap and 5 minutes prior to going to bed at night. Lie in bed—take a deep breath—exhale slowly. Close eyes. Breathe slowly. I am on an island. No stress. No one is around me. A gentle breeze—warm sunlight. Nothing else matters—for that minute.

13. **Complexion**: Blemished with acne on chin, upper neck, cheeks. **Action Plan**: Call dermatologist tomorrow (list phone number) for appointment. Don't pick or squeeze pimples.

14. **Sun damage**: Mild—Little wrinkles, no precancers, but face feels rough and looks worn from all these nights up with the baby. And there's the problem of acne. **Action Plan**: Avoid foundation makeup. Call tomorrow for appointment with dermatologist (number) for appointment to acne treatment and to discuss possibility of facial peels. Wear sunscreen at least SPF 30.

15. **Skin Aging**: Most due to sun exposure. **Action Plan**: Wear sunscreen at least SPF 30.

16. **Bad Habits**: Picking at acne spots; frowning, not wearing sunscreen. **Action Plan**: Don't pick, don't frown, do wear sunscreen.

17. **Goals**: Sure, I'd love to look like a movie star, but I guess what I really want is to look like a healthy, rested, happy person. Like the person my husband Mark married. **Action Plan**: follow the guidelines for good skin care—stick to the basics. Build upon the basics of skin care with a little makeup—lipstick, loose powder, blush, mascara—but keep the look natural. Exercise regularly, eat balanced diet, take time to relax and have fun. Note: see primary care physician (phone number) for annual check-up.

Summary Plan for Jennifer

- Buy SPF 30 sunscreen, use daily; wear hats and sunglasses when in sun.
- Buy Dove For Sensitive Skin for washing face. Buy Sal Ac Wash for washing oily areas. Buy Moisturel Lotion for use on dry areas.
- Stress-reducing exercise at kid's naptime and at bedtime. Lie in bed—take a deep breath—exhale slowly. Close eyes. Breathe slowly. I am on an island. No stress. No one is around me. A gentle breeze—warm sunlight.
- Avoid putting perfume on skin. Can dab on clothing.

- 15 minute nap when kids taking nap. Plan to go to bed by 9 pm. Call maid service for once every two week deep cleaning service.
- Buy exercise tape. 15 minutes in the living room each morning after children are fed and while they are busy playing with toys.
- Balanced diet, no snacking.
- Discuss with Mark (husband) sharing responsibilities with the children before he goes to work or after he is home. Call babysitter to schedule for Saturday nights for next month.
- Call dermatologist tomorrow (phone number) for appointment to discuss acne treatment and possibility of facial peels. Don't pick or squeeze pimples.
- Avoid foundation makeup.
- Don't pick, don't frown.
- Stick to the basics—Dove Soap, Moisturel Lotion, Sunscreen SPF 30. Add lipstick, loose powder, blush, mascara—keep the look natural.
- See primary care physician (phone number) for annual check-up.

A Plan for Carole

I'm only 32, but already my skin is starting to wear out. I've got little crinkles around my eyes, dark circles under my eyes, and a frown line between my eyebrows. I've got this redness on my cheeks and around my nose—someone said that I probably have rosacea. Plus I've got these large pores. I'm in important meetings at work, and it's really embarrassing for my face to look like this. I used to have great skin. I need to do something!

—Carole, age 32

1. **Skin Type**: Type III: Sometimes burn, usually tan, white to olive skin, brown hair, and brown eyes. **Action Plan**: Use SPF 15 or greater.
2. **Skin oiliness**: Oily. **Action Plan**: Purpose Soap for washing face. Salicylic acid wash for excess oiliness and to tighten pores.
3. **Mood**: Usually good. I'm just very tired and that sometimes makes me moody. But sometimes I do get really depressed. **Action Plan**: Get adequate rest. Seven or eight hours sleep. Call psychologist or psychiatrist to make appointment for consultation for moodiness and depression.
4. **Sunscreen**: Never. **Action Plan**: Wear sunscreen SPF 15.
5. **Perfumed Products**: I use perfumed soap. My face does itch sometimes. **Action Plan**: Discontinue perfumed soap. Use Purpose Soap.
6. **Health**: Good health, but very tired. I'm single and dating. I used to be able to stay out late and still go to work the next morning. Now I really drag through the day if I'm out late the night before. **Action Plan**: Get at least seven or eight hours of sleep per night. Call primary care physician for annual checkup.

7. **Exercise**: Never exercise. Too busy. Too tired. **Action Plan**: Join health club. Exercise half an hour at lunchtime every day.

8. **Weight**: Weight is OK, but I never really sit down and eat a meal unless I'm out to dinner with someone. But I'm out of shape—I get out of breath easily, and I have this constant cough—but that's probably from smoking. **Action Plan**: Balanced diet. Small portions OK but keep diet balanced. No fast foods. Call primary care physician (number) for exam and to help with plan to stop smoking.

9. **Appetite**: Bad when depressed, OK at other times. **Action Plan**: Schedule appointment with primary care physician (phone number). Schedule appointment with psychologist or psychiatrist (phone number).

10. **Happiness**: Sometimes. **Action Plan**: Call psychologist or psychiatrist to schedule appointment to talk about the problems and develop a plan to address the situations.

11. **Sleep**: less than five hours. **Action Plan**: Go to bed by 10 pm. Turn the phone off. Go to sleep. Confine staying out late to Friday or Saturday nights.

12. **Relaxation**: No time to relax during the day. **Action Plan**: Take a 15 minute break in the morning and in the afternoon for relaxation. Close office door, or find a quiet place at work. Stop—take a deep breath—exhale slowly. Close eyes. Breathe slowly. I am on an island. No stress. No one around me. A gentle breeze—warm sunlight.

13. **Complexion**: Ruddy on cheeks and nose. **Action Plan**: Possible rosacea—schedule appointment with dermatologist (list number) for diagnosis and treatment. Wear sunscreen.

14. **Sun Damage**: Mild—Little wrinkles, no precancers. **Action Plan**: wear sunscreen SPF 15. Avoid foundation makeup. Appointment with dermatologist to consider facial peel.

15. **Skin Aging**: Most due to sun exposure. Frown line between eyebrows and crinkles at sides of eyes can be treated with Botox. **Action Plan**: Wear sunscreen SPF 15. Make appointment with dermatologist to discuss possible Botox treatment.

16. **Bad Habits**: Wearing lots of foundation makeup, trying new products all the time; not removing makeup before going to bed. **Action Plan**: Stop doing these things.

17. **Goals**: Sure, I'd like to look like a movie star. I'd be happy all the time then. **Action Plan**: See a psychologist or psychiatrist first (phone number) to treat depression. Also see a dermatologist (phone number) to diagnose and treat the facial redness. See primary care physician for physical exam (phone number). Call to make these appointments. Use Purpose Soap for washing face; Moisturel Lotion for dryness, SalAc Wash for oiliness. Use a little makeup—lipstick, loose powder, blush,

mascara—keep the look natural. Join the gym and set up a daily exercise plan. Enlist a personal trainer to help. After seeing a psychologist or psychiatrist, reconsider goals. If still want to look like a movie star, make appointment with plastic surgeon for evaluation and consultation. Eat a balanced diet. Don't focus on plastic surgery as something that will change mood and bring happiness. Depression needs to be treated by a psychologist or psychiatrist. *Then* consider cosmetic treatments and/or plastic surgery.

Summary Plan for Carole

- Use Purpose Soap for washing face. Salicylic acid wash for excess oiliness and to tighten pores. Use Moisturel Lotion for any dryness. Use Sunscreen with SPF 15 or greater. Avoid foundation makeup.
- Get seven or eight hours sleep. Go to bed by 10 pm. Turn the phone off. Go to sleep. Confine staying out late to Friday or Saturday nights.
- Call psychologist or psychiatrist to make appointment for consultation for moodiness and depression.
- Call dermatologist (phone number) for appointment to treat facial redness, to discuss facial peels to tighten pores, and to discuss possible Botox treatment for wrinkles.
- Avoid perfumed soap.
- Call primary care physician for annual checkup and to help with plan to stop smoking.
- Join health club. Exercise half an hour at lunchtime every day. Hire personal trainer.
- Eat balanced diet. No fast foods.
- Take a 15 minute break in the morning and in the afternoon for relaxation. Close office door, or find a quiet place at work. Stop—take a deep breath—exhale slowly. Close eyes. Breathe slowly. I am on an island. No stress. No one around me. A gentle breeze—warm sunlight.
- Stop trying new products all the time.
- Remove all makeup before going to bed.
- After consultation with psychologist or psychiatrist to treat depression, make appointment with plastic surgery to consider options for appearance.

A Plan for Miriam

I'm 65 and at a wonderful stage in life. My husband and I have retired to a beautiful, sunny place in the South, in a community full of great people. I was amazed at how youthful many of the retirees look, and then I discovered that they have had all sorts of wonderful treatments by a dermatologist in the area. Some I know have had plastic surgery. I'm very happy with my life, but

I would love to find out what would be appropriate for my skin to take off some years!

—*Miriam, age 65*

1. **Skin Type**: Type II (Usually burn, sometimes tan, have white skin, blond hair, blue or green eyes.). **Action Plan**: use sunscreen with SPF 30, wear hats and sunglasses when in sun.
2. **Skin oiliness**: dry. **Action Plan**: Use a mild unscented soap such as Dove or Cetaphil. Pat dry and apply a small amount of Purpose Lotion with SPF 30.
3. **Mood**: Happy almost all of the time. **Action Plan**: Continue happy mood. Try to cheer up others. Think happy thoughts—a happy face is a beautiful face.
4. **Sunscreen**: Always now, but I didn't when I was younger—that's why I have all these wrinkles now. **Action Plan**: Always wear a sunscreen to prevent photoaging and to reduce the risk of skin cancer.
5. **Perfumed Products**: I use perfumed soaps and lotions and apply scented bath powder. I have been itching on my legs recently. **Action Plan**: Perfumed products can irritate skin. Try leaving off dark hose to see if that is the cause of itching legs. If that doesn't clear the problem, leave off the perfumed soaps, lotions, and bath powder. Can dab a little perfume on clothing.
6. **Health**: I'm fortunate to have good health—am not aware of anything wrong, but it has been awhile since I've had a checkup. **Action Plan**: Call primary care physician for checkup.
7. **Exercise**: I play golf occasionally with my friends. Otherwise I don't have a regular exercise plan. **Action Plan**: Have a daily exercise program and stick to it—join gym, plan daily early morning walk. Wear sunscreen.
8. **Weight**: Overweight. Since I turned 60, I haven't been able to keep the weight off. **Action Plan**: Call primary care physician (phone number) or nutritionist (phone number) to start a sensible diet.
9. **Appetite**: Too good. **Action Plan**: Plan exercise program, stay away from the refrigerator. Plan balanced diet with small portions.
10. **Happiness**: Almost always, thank goodness. **Action Plan**: Continue enjoying life.
11. **Sleep**: Eight hours—I need this to feel good during the day. **Action Plan**: Continue getting adequate sleep.
12. **Relaxation**: Yes. I get a wonderful massage once a week. And now that I'm retired I can take time to sit and read a book. I'd like to try some aromatherapy that I've read about. **Action Plan**: Continue taking time to relax. Continue massages. Try aromatherapy—there are lots of ways to relax.

13. **Complexion**: Wrinkled with sun damage, with patchy dark spots. **Action Plan**: Protect skin with mild soap, moisturizer if skin is dry, and sunscreen, at least SPF 45 or greater. See dermatologist to make sure that dark spots are benign and not skin cancers or precancers. Ask dermatologist about creams to help fade sun spots. Discuss with dermatologist the possibility of chemical peels to help fade these spots.

14. **Sun Damage**: Severe wrinkling, photoaging, skin sagging. **Action Plan**: Have regular check-ups for detection and treatment of precancers or skin cancers, and wear sunscreen at all times

15. **Skin Aging**: Severe intrinsic aging as well as photoaging. **Action Plan**: Consult with dermatologist or plastic surgeon to formulate plan for erasing wrinkles, lifting skin, firming skin. Ask the physician to discuss the following:

   – Restylane injections to fill in deep wrinkles above lips and between nose and mouth.
   – Intense pulsed light or Fraxel treatments to firm up skin and give a more youthful appearance and to remove tiny blood vessels on face.
   – Botox to treat crows' feet, forehead wrinkles, and wrinkles between the eyebrows.
   – Blepharoplasty to remove eyelid droop
   – Face lift to tighten and lift skin.
   – Chemical peels to smooth facial skin

16. **Bad Habits**: Wearing lots of foundation makeup. **Action Plan**: Do not wear foundation—it clogs pores and accentuates wrinkles. Use a little blush and eye makeup and some loose powder—buy new, fresh products.

17. **Goals**: Ten years younger and a healthy, happy person. **Action Plan**: Schedule appointment with dermatologist (phone number) or plastic surgeon (phone number) to formulate a Transformation Plan: consider facial peels, facial resurfacing, intense pulsed light treatments, microdermabrasion, Fraxel treatments, or Sculptra or Restylane injections, face lifts. Follow good skin care of mild soap, unscented moisturizer, sunscreen. Schedule appointment with primary care physician (phone number) for a check-up. Plan exercise schedule, plan balanced diet, take time to relax and have fun.

Summary Plan for Miriam

- Use sunscreen with at least SPF 30, wear hats and sunglasses when in sun.
- Use a mild unscented soap such as Dove or Cetaphil. Pat dry and apply a small amount of Purpose Lotion with SPF 30.
- Think happy thoughts.

- Stop wearing dark hose to see if that is the cause of itching legs. Leave off perfumed soaps, lotions, and bath powder. Can dab a little perfume on clothing.
- Call primary care physician for checkup.
- Have daily exercise program and stick to it—join gym, plan daily early morning walk. Stay away from refrigerator. Plan balanced diet with small portions.
- Call primary care physician (phone number) for check-up and to start a sensible diet.
- Continue eight hours sleep each night.
- Continue taking time to relax. Continue massages. Try aromatherapy.
- Schedule appointment with dermatologist (phone number) for full skin exam. Plan regular checkups for detection and treatment of precancers or skin cancers.
- Consult with dermatologist (phone number) or plastic surgeon (phone number) to formulate plan for erasing wrinkles, lifting skin, firming skin. Ask the physician to discuss all options.
- Avoid foundation makeup. Use a little blush and eye makeup and some loose powder—buy new, fresh products.
- Schedule appointment with dermatologist (phone number) or plastic surgeon (phone number) to formulate a Transformation Plan: consider facial peels, facial resurfacing, intense pulsed light treatments, microdermabrasion, Fraxel treatments, or Sculptra or Restylane injections, face lifts. Discuss all options.

Now it's time to make your own Action Plan and, if necessary, to develop with your dermatologist or plastic surgeon your Transformation Plan. Be brave, be bold, but most of all, take action!

PART IV

SKIN PROBLEMS

CHAPTER 15

WHAT YOU NEED TO KNOW ABOUT SKIN CANCER

I've lived in the sun all my life. Now that I've turned 30, I'm getting these spots on my arms and legs and my face. I'm not sure what not to worry about and what might be skin cancer.

—Kristin, age 38

It's important to have a regular skin exam, especially if you grew up spending a lot of time in the sun. Removing skin cancers can result in scars, sometimes disfiguring, but they must be removed to prevent even larger scars and/or death.

A tiny spot on the skin can be simply a harmless "sun spot" or can be a deadly skin cancer. It is important not only to have an annual skin exam but to also conduct your own monthly self examination. It *can* be a matter of life or death!

THE SUN AND YOUR SKIN

I just can't believe that sun is bad for skin. It feels so good to lie out—and I feel so healthy! Sure, I know it's supposed to cause skin cancer—but isn't some sun good for you? Don't we need Vitamin D or something from sunshine?

—Donald, age 45

Sunshine feels good on skin, and being outdoors on a sunny day can make you feel cheerful and healthy. Sun does good things for skin, but it also does bad things. Moderation is the answer—and that's not lying out for a shorter period of time. That's wearing sunscreen and protecting from sun—you'll still get enough sunlight but hopefully not too much to burn or increase your risk of skin cancers.

Ultraviolet radiation from the sun penetrates skin and can reach not only the skin surface to cause sunburn, but can also get into skin cells to damage the DNA found there. When DNA is damaged, cells have a mechanism for cutting out and repairing the damaged DNA. But sometimes the damage is so much that the cell is overwhelmed and begins to divide before the DNA can be repaired.

The new cells carry the same damaged DNA and will in turn divide in a vicious cycle of damaged cells giving birth to more damaged cells. Such uncontrolled cell growth results in skin cancer.

ACTINIC KERATOSES

I play tennis at the club every Tuesday and Thursday, and usually have a game on Sunday afternoon. I've been wearing a sunscreen with an SPF 8, but I've been getting these rough pink spots that won't go away on my cheeks and nose.
—Deborah, age 34

Actinic keratoses[1] are common precancerous lesions that occur most frequently on fair-skinned individuals with a history of sun exposure. They are rough, sandpaper-like spots often found on the forehead, temples, ears, nose, cheeks, forearms, hands, and on balding scalps. They can also be found on the upper chest and upper back. They may be red, white, pink, or tan. If left untreated, some of these may change over time into squamous cell skin carcinomas. Actinic keratoses can be treated in the dermatologist's office with liquid nitrogen or at home with a cream such as imiquimod or 5 percent fluorouracil applied for several weeks.

If liquid nitrogen is used for treatment, the dermatologist will either spray it on the precancer or dip a cotton-tipped swab in liquid nitrogen and apply. There is some stinging at the time of application that usually resolves in a few minutes. During the next several minutes the precancer will become bright pink and puffy, and over the next week or two it will become crusty and scaly. Blistering of the area may occur. Around the second or third week the crust and scale will come off, and there should be no more spot. If there's any part of the spot left, it is important to return to the dermatologist for further treatment.

Topical medications, such as imiquimod (Aldara), 5-flourouracil (Efudex), or diclofenac (Solaraze) gel, can be effective in getting rid of actinic keratoses. This requires diligent application and quite a bit of inflammation and irritation can occur over the treatment period. Imiquimod is applied twice a week at night for a couple of months. Efudex is applied twice a day for three to six weeks. Solaraze is applied twice a day for two to three months. One advantage of topical treatment is that the medication does treat lesions that are not yet clinically evident.

Use a sunscreen, a hat, and other protective clothing when you are outdoors. SPF 8 isn't enough! Use at least SPF 15, and if you are out in the sun any length of time, use at least SPF 30.

I never go into the sun, so I don't have to worry about wearing sun screen.
—Babs, age 38

Wrong! Unless you hide in a closet all day you do have sun exposure. And remember, sun damage is cumulative. That means that the sun exposure that you get now, however small, adds to the sun exposure in your earlier years and continues to increase your risk of developing precancers and skin cancers.

Photodynamic therapy (PDT), another treatment for precancers, calls on the power of light to destroy precancerous cells. A "photosensitizing agent"— something that makes skin more sensitive to light—is applied to the skin. The precancers preferentially absorb the photosensitizing agent. When the skin is then exposed to a certain wavelength of light, the precancers are destroyed. This treatment, though usually effective, can be slightly painful during the first 5 minutes or so of the 15 minute exposure to the light.

DANGER SIGNS OF SKIN CANCER: KNOW YOUR A, B, C, D, E'S!

I was born with a lot of moles, and I keep getting more. I got this from my father's side of the family. My father died of melanoma, so I know that I need to be careful. Some of my moles have jagged edges and some are very large. What should I know about moles to reduce my chances of dying from melanoma too?

—Andre, age 24

Moles ("nevi" in dermatology language, or "nevus" if a single mole) have different sizes, shapes, and colors. It is important to recognize danger signs in moles. Any mole that bleeds, hurts, or itches, or changes in color or shape should be examined immediately by a dermatologist. A full-skin examination at least once a year is very important, or more often if any abnormal moles are found. Andre should see a dermatologist right away. If he has abnormal moles, he should be checked every six months.

Danger signs include a mole that is irregular (asymmetric) in shape, a mole with an irregular (jagged or indented) border, a mole containing different colors (especially a very dark color), a large mole (as large as the eraser on the end of a pencil), or a new mole (an "evolving" mole). These are some of the characteristics of melanoma, the most dangerous type of skin cancer.

Dysplastic Moles

I've had this mole all of my life but lately it has been getting darker. Is this anything to worry about?

—Brian, age 26

It is very important to be examined by a dermatologist if any moles change. Your dermatologist will determine whether any of your moles should be removed. If so, the moles that are removed will be sent to the laboratory for

---

DANGER SIGNS IN MOLES

A: Asymmetry: A mole develops a "lopsided" appearance. If you were to cut the mole in half, one side would look different from the other

B: Border Irregularity: A mole develops a jagged border

C: Color Changes: A mole develops different colors in it—this may be the development of different shades of brown, black, red, or blue, or the mole may just be getting very dark

D: Diameter: Enlargement: A mole starts growing and reaches the size of an eraser on a pencil

E: Evolving Mole: A new mole developing

In addition to the A, B, C, D, E danger signs in moles, be sure to see your dermatologist if a mole becomes itchy, bleeds, or changes in any other way.

---

microscopic examination. Even if an irregular mole turns out not to be a melanoma, it may be "dysplastic"[2] (atypical). Dysplastic moles have a higher risk of turning into melanoma. If you have a melanoma or a dysplastic mole, you will need to be followed by your dermatologist on a regular basis to check for the development of any additional moles with abnormalities.

Melanoma

My favorite uncle had a mole for as long as he could remember. It began to get darker, but he didn't pay much attention to it, because it had "always" been

---

WHAT HAPPENS WHEN YOU HAVE A MOLE EXCISED

- The doctor will wash the mole and surrounding area with an antiseptic solution such as Hibiclens or Betadine.
- The doctor will inject local anesthesia such as Lidocaine around and under the mole. This will sting but lasts only a few seconds.
- The mole will be excised with a blade. This part should not be painful because the area will be numb from the anesthesia.
- The mole will be sent to a laboratory for examination.
- If the area excised was large and/or deep, the doctor will suture the area excised. You will need to return in a couple of weeks for suture removal.
- The doctor will tell you how to take care of the excision site. This will usually involve keeping the area dry overnight. You are usually allowed to bathe the area gently the next day. You will need to apply an antibiotic ointment or Vaseline to the affected area twice a day. If the area becomes crusty, you can clean it gently with a Q-tip dipped in hydrogen peroxide.

WHAT HAPPENS IF YOUR DERMATOLOGIST FINDS A MOLE SUSPICIOUS FOR MELANOMA

Your dermatologist will excise the mole and send it to the pathology laboratory for evaluation. If the mole turns out to be a melanoma, more skin will need to be removed around the excision site to make certain that the melanoma has been completely removed.

The pathology report will be important in predicting the outcome. If the melanoma is still in the upper portion (epidermis) of the skin and has not penetrated the lower portion (dermis), the outcome is expected to be excellent. If the melanoma has penetrated the dermis, the outcome is related to the how far down in the skin the melanoma has spread and whether it has spread to other areas. Further tests will be necessary depending upon the depth of the melanoma.

there. One day it began to bleed, and he put a bandaid over it, thinking that he must have scratched it. Afterwards it seemed to always be irritated, so he just kept a bandaid on it. It was in the V of his neck. I was just a young child at the time, and I remember crawling into his lap to read a book and seeing the bandaid—it seemed to always be there. He became sick with what he thought was pneumonia. He was usually a healthy person—didn't have time for doctors, but he had to see one this time. The doctor put him in the hospital. He died a week later from melanoma.

Who would have thought that something as small as a mole could kill my uncle. Unbelievable! Those were the days before skin cancer screenings and public awareness of melanoma.

Melanoma is a cancerous mole. It can be deadly if not removed in time. It is of utmost importance that you see your dermatologist immediately if you have a mole with bleeding, itching, changes in shape, development of a jagged border, changes in color (including appearance of different shades of brown or black) or increase in size,[3] or if you see a new mole developing or a mole changing in any way.

Even if you don't notice any changes in your moles, your skin should be checked once a year by a dermatologist to make certain that no abnormal changes have occurred.

The incidence of melanoma is increasing at an alarming rate.[4] Blistering sunburns—especially those in your childhood—can increase the risk of developing melanoma.[5] Wear sunscreen and protective clothing and protect your children likewise from the sun. Do not use tanning beds.

What Happens When You Have a Skin Biopsy?

If you have a skin biopsy, the dermatologist will inject a small amount of anesthesia such as Lidocaine into the skin to "numb" the area to be biopsied. The doctor will then surgically remove a small piece of skin and send it to a laboratory for evaluation. You will be instructed to keep the biopsied area dry overnight and to apply antibacterial ointment such as Bacitracin twice a day for a couple of weeks until the area heals. If the doctor puts in sutures to close the biopsy site, you will be asked to come back in five to seven days for removal of the sutures if the biopsy site is on the face, or in 10 to 14 days if the biopsy site is elsewhere on the body.

OTHER SKIN CANCERS

Basal cell carcinoma and squamous cell carcinoma are two types of skin cancers commonly seen. It is important to see your dermatologist if a new growth appears or if a sore does not heal.

Basal Cell Carcinoma

There's this little pink, shiny bump on my nose that just doesn't go away. It's been there about two months and doesn't bother me except that it's still there. I tend to burn easily in the sun. Could it be from sun damage or something?
　　　　　　　　　　　　　　　　　　　　　　　　　—Marilyn, age 42.

The most common type of skin cancer in the age range of 40 to 50 years old is basal cell carcinoma.[6] It can occur in other age groups as well.

Sun exposure at present or in the past greatly increases the risk of developing basal cell carcinoma. This skin cancer commonly appears as a pink, pearly papule in a sun-exposed area. It can eventually develop an ulcerated center, and tiny blood vessels (telangectasia) can sometimes be seen on the surface of the papule. Basal cell carcinoma on the face can sometimes first appear as a flesh-colored papule. These skin cancers can also appear in other forms, including a whitish patch that looks like a scar, and a pink patch with a slight sheen.

Fair-skinned individuals have a greater risk of developing basal cell carcinomas than those with dark skin. Patients with a rare genetic condition called basal cell nevus syndrome develop hundreds of basal cell carcinomas over their lifetime in sun exposed and non-sun exposed areas.

See your dermatologist once a year for a full skin exam, and immediately if new growths occur, so that biopsy of suspicious growths can be performed. Basal cell skin cancers need to be excised to prevent spread to deeper tissues and bone. Some of the worst pictures in dermatology text books are of patients who have

---

How Does a Biopsy Differ From an Excision?

The steps are the same. The reason is different. An excision attempts to move an entire growth. A biopsy takes only a piece of the growth or a rash for diagnostic purposes—to find out what it is but not necessarily to take it all out at that time.

---

lost a nose, an ear, or part of their face and scalp because they let a basal cell carcinoma go too long without seeing their doctor.

Squamous Cell Carcinoma

I have this crusted spot on the back of my hand that seems to be getting bigger. I thought it was a wart at first, but it seems to have a lot of scale and crust. Is this anything to worry about?

—John, age 62

Squamous cell carcinoma[7] can develop in actinic keratoses and at sites of injury, such as in burns, scars, and areas of sun damage. It can also develop in skin areas that have been exposed to X-Ray treatment. Sun exposure increases the risk of developing squamous cell carcinoma. This skin cancer can also develop in areas without a history of injury. It occurs most often in persons age 60 or older but can be found in any age group. It can look like a wart, an ulcerated nodule, or any other non-healing lesion.

Squamous cell carcinomas have a greater potential than basal cell carcinomas to spread to other areas through the blood stream (metastasize), and like other

---

Remember

- Actinic keratoses are precancerous lesions. See your dermatologist for treatment.
- Malignant melanoma is a potentially deadly form of skin cancer. See your dermatologist for any new or changing mole.
- Basal cell carcinoma and squamous cell carcinoma are common forms of skin cancer.
- See your dermatologist immediately if a sore does not heal after a few weeks, if a new growth appears and persists, and if any spot bleeds or changes color or size.

skin cancers, should be excised to remove the lesion entirely. Sun protection is very important. This form of skin cancer can be a significant and recurring problem in patients who are taking medications that suppress the immune system.

Most skin cancers can be satisfactorily treated if detected early enough. See your dermatologist at least once a year for a full skin exam and any time a spot changes or a new spot develops.

THE SKIN SELF-EXAM

Check your skin from top to bottom, front to back, at least once a month (Figure 15.1). Here's how:

- Get a big hand-held mirror and a magnifying glass from the drugstore.
- Strip naked and stand in front of a full length mirror.
- Make sure that you are in a well-lit area so that you can see your skin well.
- Have a notepad for jotting down anything that worries you or that has changed since your last exam.

Let's get started:

HERE'S WHAT YOU WILL BE LOOKING FOR

- Moles that are asymmetrical, have border irregularities, color changes, or a diameter as large or greater than a pencil eraser.
- Non-healing sores.
- Pink shiny bumps, especially in sun exposed areas, that are not going away.
- Any other skin changes—no change is too small to have checked by your dermatologist—better to check now if in doubt than be sorry later.

See your dermatologist if you discover any changes during your exam. It is important to have a "baseline skin exam" and at least a yearly skin exam thereafter. This will give you a chance to "know your skin" and to determine what changes are normal and which are not. Having regular exams, doing a monthly self-exam, and seeing your dermatologist if anything changes can save your life!

THE FULL SKIN SELF-EXAM

- **SCALP**: Start from the top: shake your hair forward and feel for any bumps in your scalp. It's also good to have a friend and/or spouse who can look through your scalp to make certain there are no dark spots that you wouldn't be able to feel.
- **FACE AND NECK**: Shake your hair back and examine your face and neck. Use the magnifying glass if your eyes aren't as sharp as they used to be.
- **CHEST, ABDOMEN**: Examine your chest, breasts, under your breasts, and your abdomen for any of these changes.
- **ARMS**: Extend your arms straight out from your side and examine. Keeping your arms straight out from your side, rotate your arms as far forward as possible—and then as far backwards as possible. Look for any of the changes listed above.
- **UNDERARMS**: Raise your arms straight up and examine under your arms. Let your eyes look carefully over your entire arms, then lower your arms to a comfortable position.
- **HANDS**: Examine each hand and each finger.
- **LEGS**: Look carefully down the full extent of your legs, turning them from one side to the other to examine the sides.
- **FEET**: Turn your back to the full-length mirror, look over your shoulder, and hold one foot up at a time to examine the bottom of each foot. If you are unsteady standing on one foot don't try this—use a stool to sit on instead and, facing the mirror, lift one foot and examine the bottom in the mirror, and then lift the other foot and examine it.
- **BACK**: Now you'll need your hand mirror. Turn your back to the full-length mirror and use your hand mirror to examine your entire back, paying special attention to sun-exposed areas such as the upper back and shoulders
- **BUTTOCKS AND LOWER LEGS**: Examine the back of each arm, and then examine your buttocks and lower legs.

Figure 15.1. Skin self-exam. [Reprinted with permission from the American Academy of Dermatology. All rights reserved.]

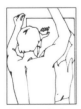 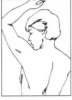 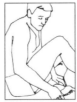 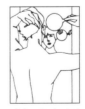 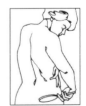

1 Examine body front and back in mirror, then right and left sides, arms raised.

2 Bend elbows, look carefully at forearms, back of upper arms, and palms.

3 Look at backs of legs and feet, spaces between toes, and soles.

4 Examine back of neck and scalp with a hand mirror. Part hair and lift.

5 Finally, check back and buttocks with a hand mirror.

CHAPTER 16

DRY SKIN, CHAPPED LIPS, AND MOTTLED SKIN

I'm from Boston and in the wintertime my skin gets so dry it cracks—especially my hands. What can I do?
—*Mary Lou, age 37*

DRY SKIN

Wintertime can be harsh on skin, especially in cold climates when the heat is on inside. The heat dries out skin just as it dries out houseplants and everything else. A humidifier can help, and applying a moisturizer after bathing is especially important to prevent evaporation of moisture from skin. Apply within the first minute after towel-drying. Mineral oil or petroleum jelly can also be helpful for chapped hands or other areas of extremely dry skin. If there are painful cracks on your fingers, apply an over-the-counter antibiotic ointment such as Bacitracin ointment to the cracks. Try applying petroleum jelly and wearing white cotton gloves (from the drugstore) overnight if your hands are especially irritated.

Dry skin ("xerosis" in dermatology terms) can also occur with age and with certain skin disorders. See your dermatologist if this condition does not improve. Irritated skin can sometimes become infected, requiring an antibiotic to clear.

DRY LIPS

My lips are cracking so much that I can't eat without their starting to bleed. I lick them to make them moist, but they just seem to get worse.
—*Leandra, age 28*

Dry lips can be caused by dry air, by reaction to lipstick, toothpaste, food, medication,[1] or by lip licking. Licking your lips will just make your lips more dry and chapped. Apply an unscented lip balm or petroleum jelly and see your dermatologist if the problem does not clear.

MOTTLED SKIN

I spent a lot of time at the beach in my teens and 20s, and I used to get the perfect tan. Now when I go play golf and I get sun on my arms and legs, my skin looks all mottled—with dark and light spots. What's happening!
                                                        —Melinda, age 42

In your 30s or 40s you may notice that you no longer tan. Instead, your skin looks speckled and splotchy and may itch after being in the sun. This is nature's way of reminding you that sun damages skin. The light spots are where the skin's pigment cells have been killed by the sun. The dark spots are where the pigment cells have tried to multiply to protect your skin from the sun.

Alas, now your skin looks much older than if you had avoided the sun. This is one of the symptoms of "photoaging" and one of the signs that your skin is at increased risk of developing skin cancers.

Apply sunscreen, wear protective clothing, and avoid sun exposure in the middle of the day. Protect your skin from the sun!

CHAPTER 17

PROBLEMS WITH HAIR AND SCALP

I'm so upset! My hair is falling out! I've been finding clumps of hair in the shower after I shampoo, and my hairbrush is always full of hair. I'm starting to see my scalp through my hair, and I don't know what to do!

—*Agnes, age 31*

THINNING HAIR

Losing hair is cause for great distress for most people. You are taking good care of your hair, but it keeps falling out! What is happening! What can you do! You don't want to go bald when you're only 30!

Many factors can contribute to thinning of hair.[1] Your hair will naturally thin in your 40s and 50s, and sometimes earlier. The amount of thinning will depend on part on the genes that you have inherited. Do the women in your family tend to have thinning hair? Think back not only to your current generation of relatives, but to your mother, your grandmother, as far back as you can. Hair loss with aging is referred to by dermatologists as "androgenic alopecia."

But there are many other causes of hair loss. One of the most common is a "resting phase" of hair growth called "telogen effluvium." Many hairs just "take a rest" and stop growing. More hair falls out than grows in. A lot of hair will be found on the hairbrush and on the shower drain after shampooing.

After a period of two or three months, but sometimes up to a year or more, normal hair growth may resume. Many stressful events can precipitate "telogen effluvium," including having a baby, undergoing surgery, and being ill. Often there's no precipitating cause—it may be due to "the natural cycle of things."

The hairs that shed during "telogen effluvium" have already gone through the active growth phase and are in the "resting" (telogen) phase of hair growth. In contrast, another type of hair loss, called "anagen effluvium" results in shedding of actively growing hairs. "Anagen effluvium" is caused by many factors, including certain medications, illnesses, and stress. By examining the loose hairs by microscope, your dermatologist can determine whether resting or actively growing hairs are shedding. This can be helpful in determining why you are losing hair and whether it is likely to regrow.

There are other reasons for hair loss. Many medications can cause hair loss. Medical problems such as abnormal thyroid conditions can result in hair loss. Irritated and flaking scalps can cause hair loss. Pulling or twisting hair or wearing it pulled back in a pony tail or braided can cause hair loss. Scalp conditions can cause hair loss—sometimes with scarring and permanent loss of hair.

A fairly common type of hair loss involves loss of hair in circular areas on the scalp. This is called "alopecia areata."[2] Eyebrows, beard, and any hair-bearing area may be affected. In fact, sometimes all hair is lost on the scalp ("alopecia totalis") or, rarely, everywhere on the body ("alopecia universalis"). The cause of alopecia areata is unknown, but it is thought that the cells that comprise part of the body's natural defense system become confused and attack the hair follicles, thinking for some reason that one's own hair follicles are foreign invaders to the body.

If you develop alopecia areata, your doctor may be able to "set things straight" by prescribing steroid creams to apply to the bald areas or by injecting steroid into those areas. Hair usually regrows over time in most cases of alopecia areata, but the condition may recur.[3]

But what about the other types of hair loss? For men and women with hair loss due to aging, there is Rogaine (minoxidil, Upjohn Co.), regular strength (2 percent) and extra strength (5 percent).[4] Rogaine helps widen blood vessels and may make some hair grow, although often these are "vellus" hairs, or "peach fuzz." Rogaine was once available only by prescription, but can now be obtained over the counter at the pharmacy.

For men there is also finasteride (Propecia[5]). Propecia is the first FDA-approved drug in pill form for hair loss (for use in males only). Propecia works by blocking a hormone called DHT that is important in male hair loss.[6] After a year of treatment with Propecia, most men with mild to moderate hair loss appear to either stop or slow hair loss or to grow more hair. Rarely, there can be side effects that include loss of sex drive, difficulty in achieving an erection, and decreased production of semen.

The bottom line is that the real solution to stopping hair loss and growing new hair just isn't out there yet. But drug companies are racing with one another to find something that will work—the demand is there, the market is there, and the first to come up with a really effective product will in truth win the golden ring.

There are also cosmetic treatments such as hair transplantation and scalp reduction that can give the appearance of having more hair. These procedures are discussed in Chapter 8.

HORMONES AND HAIR LOSS

Can menopause affect hair loss? I have a lot of shedding of hair and my hair is now much thinner. This started several years ago when I started going through menopause.

—*Casey, age 51*

Hormones play a role in hair growth and hair loss. It's not uncommon for women going through menopause, or women on birth control pills, to begin to lose hair.

Fortunately we do not normally shed all of our hair at one time. Instead, each hair is in its own cycle of growth, resting, and falling out. As a hair falls out, a new hair begins to grow, and the anagen phase takes over again in that hair follicle. About 90 percent of hairs are usually in the anagen (growth) phase at any one time, while about 10 percent are in the telogen (resting) phase. In this way, we maintain a full head of hair while we go through the process of shedding and regrowing hairs.

Since hormones play a role in stimulating hair growth, changes in hormones can throw out of balance the normal proportion of hairs in the anagen phase to hairs in the telogen phase. Remember that some shedding is natural. In fact, losing around 100 hairs during one day is normal.

Other factors that can affect hair loss include illness, physical stress, Vitamin A derivatives, cholesterol-lowering medications, and certain high blood pressure medications (beta blockers). If your hair is thinning, see your physician to discuss possible underlying causes of your hair loss.

SEBORRHEIC DERMATITIS

My scalp is flaking! I can't wear anything dark, because the dandruff looks like snow on my shoulders. What can I do!

—Patricia, age 28

Seborrheic dermatitis[7] is a common skin condition. Many people are familiar with dandruff, a characteristic of this condition. The scalp also may be itchy, and thick crust may form. "Cradle cap," where baby's scalp has thick crust, is a form of seborrheic dermatitis in infants. Treatment for "cradle cap" is discussed in Chapter 9.

In adults there may also be redness and scaling around the nose, in the eyebrows, along the hairline, behind the ears, and in the ears.

If you have seborrheic dermatitis, your doctor may recommend a medicated, over-the-counter shampoo such as Nizoral Shampoo[8] (2 percent ketoconazole), Sebulex Shampoo[9] (2 percent sulfa, 2 percent salicylic acid), Selsun Shampoo[10] (2.5 percent selenium sulfide lotion), or Head and Shoulders[11] (1 percent pyrithione zinc). Leave the shampoo on for five to ten minutes before rinsing so that it will have time to treat your scalp. If there is a lot of crust or scale, your doctor may prescribe an oil (Dermasmoothe) to apply to your scalp at night and wash out the next morning. If you are not allergic to peanuts, you can apply peanut oil at night and wash out the next morning. Such "oil treatments" will help remove thick scale.

For seborrheic dermatitis involving the face and other areas, your doctor may prescribe an anti-yeast cream such as Nizoral[12] (ketoconazole) Cream.

Be sure to see your physician if you have flaking of your scalp or redness of your face. There are other conditions that can cause flaking of the scalp and redness of the face. See your doctor to confirm the reason for these symptoms.

FOLLICULITIS

I train for marathons—wear these tights in the winter that make my legs feel and look good—until I take them off. There are little bumps everywhere on my legs! I know what razor burn looks like, but I'm getting them on my arms and chest, too, and I sure don't shave there! Why am I getting these!

—Carol Lynn, age 25

Hair follicles can become irritated for a variety of reasons, resulting in "folliculitis." This can happen from rubbing, sweating, shaving, or any other type of friction. Excessive sweating can cause irritation of the follicles. The result is tiny red bumps around individual hair follicles.

If you take a magnifying glass and look at one of the bumps, there will be a tiny hair protruding from the middle of the bump. Joggers and weight lifters often have this problem on their chest and back as a result of excessive sweating. Shaving legs ("razor burn") or wearing tight pants and jeans that rub hairs on the legs can also result in folliculitis.

Sometimes folliculitis is caused by bacteria that get down the hair shaft and irritate the hair follicle. For example, "hot tub folliculitis"[13] can result after an otherwise wonderful soak in a hot tub. Why? Pseudomonas, a bacteria that can infect hair follicles, likes to live in wet environments such as in hot tubs.

If you have red bumps on your legs or anywhere, see your dermatologist. There are many other types of "red bumps" that can occur on skin, and you need an accurate diagnosis by a trained physician. If you have folliculitis, your dermatologist may prescribe a salicylic acid or benzoyl peroxide wash, a topical antibiotic, a moisturizer, or an oral antibiotic, depending upon the degree and location of the folliculitis.

HIRSUTISM

I have too much dark hair on my face and chest. It's on my upper lip, on my chin, and around my nipples. This began when I turned thirteen. What's going on?

—Lynn, age 28

Hirsutism is excessive hair growth on a woman's face or body that creates a pattern of hair growth similar to that of a male. The excessive hair growth may be in the mustache and beard area, around the nipples, and sometimes in a line down the abdomen. The hairs are usually coarse and more like scalp hairs rather than the fine, almost invisible hairs normally seen sometimes in these areas.

In hirsutism, hair follicles are overstimulated by excessive androgen hormones, such as testosterone. Androgen hormones are the primary sex hormones in men. They are usually found in low levels in women. Sometimes excessive male hormones in women are caused by abnormalities in the ovaries, the adrenal glands, or the pituitary gland of the brain. Sometimes they may be caused by certain medications.

If you have excessive dark hair growth on your face or other parts of your body, especially if your menstrual cycles are irregular or if the excessive hair growth is a recent development, be sure to see your physician for examination and testing for hormone irregularities. There are ways to remove excessive hair, but the underlying cause should be determined.

THINNING EYEBROWS

My eyebrows are thinning. I have to use more and more eyebrow pencil to make my eyebrows look like they are still there. Is this just because I'm growing older?
—Madeline, age 52

Eyebrow hair, as well as scalp hair, can thin with aging. But there are also other causes to consider. Vigorous use of an eyebrow pencil or rubbing or scratching eyebrows can also increase hair loss in eyebrows. Gentle treatment of eyebrows is important. If you use an eyebrow pencil or brush, be sure to use light strokes and do not rub.

Certain medical conditions, such as alopecia areata, and certain medications can also cause loss of eyebrows. Loss of hair on the outer one-third of the eyebrow ("Hertzoge's sign") is sometimes associated with low thyroid conditions (hypothyroid) or endocrine imbalances. Eczema can cause loss of eyebrow hair, usually from scratching. See your physician for any underlying medical condition that might be causing loss of eyebrow hair.

CHAPTER 18

ACNE, ROSACEA, AND OTHER FACIAL BLEMISHES

ACNE

I'm in my thirties and all of a sudden it's like I'm a teenager again! My face and neck are breaking out with acne, of all things—and even worse than in my teen years—the bumps are big and deep and sore. What's happening!?
—Carlotta, age 32.

Acne[1] is a common teen problem that can also occur in the 20s and 30s or even later in life. There are many different types of acne and degrees of severity. Often there are inflammatory (pink) papules, pustules (pimples), comedones (blackheads and whiteheads), painful cysts, and scarring.[2, 3] These signs of acne usually occur on the face and can also involve the back, the upper chest, and the upper arms.

What causes acne? Hormones, thickened walls of sebaceous ducts, and bacteria play important roles in development of acne:

1. Hormones that are particularly active during teen years, and also in later years, stimulate sebaceous (oil) glands in skin to produce an abundance of sebum (a mixture of oil and wax). Sebum tries to get to the surface of skin through specialized channels called sebaceous ducts. Sebum plays a normal role in moisturizing the skin surface, but when too much is produced, it has a hard time getting through the ducts.
2. To make matters worse, the walls of the ducts become thickened, blocking travel of sebum upwards to the skin surface, causing those deep, painful acne cysts.
3. Bacteria take advantage of this blockage, and go to work on the sebum, breaking it down into components that cause inflammation (redness) of skin. The end result is sore, painful, inflamed acne cysts.

I always thought that chocolate, fried foods, nuts, and other foods caused acne —or at least made it worse.
—Sarah, age 43

Hormones have more of an effect on acne flares than foods. But if your acne seems to flare after eating certain foods, avoid those foods.

I've got a big event coming up next month, and I look horrible. Not only is my face broken out, but I've got painful acne bumps on my back and chest. What can I do?

—*Rachael, age 36*

If you have acne without the deep cysts, your dermatologist may prescribe topical treatment, which may consist of a topical antibiotic to apply in the morning and a topical retinoid or other agent to apply at night. Topical antibiotics that may be prescribed include Cleocin T[4] (clindamycin phosphate topical solution, gel, or lotion), erythromycin gel[5], ointment, or solution, or topical sulfonamide such as Klaron[6] Lotion (sodium sulfacetamide). Topical retinoids include Retin-A,[7] Micro and Avita[8] Cream or Gel, and Tazorac[9] (tazarotene gel). Other topical agents used for treatment of acne include Azelex[10] (azelaic acid cream or gel) and Differin[11] (adapaline gel, cream, or solution). Benzoyl peroxide[12] washes and gels such as Brevoxyl-4 (or Brevoxyl-8)[13] Cleansing Lotion, Wash, or Gel can also be helpful. Be sure to rinse your skin well after using such washes. They contain benzoyl peroxide, which can stain towels and clothes.

If inflammatory (red, inflamed) cysts are present, your dermatologist may prescribe oral antibiotics.[14]

I've tried everything for acne, but nothing seems to work. My doctors have prescribed creams and pills for years, but I've still got these painful cysts and scars all over my face, my back, and my arms.

—*Bobby, age 19*

In cases of severe, nodular, and scarring acne where other treatments have failed, your dermatologist may discuss treatment with isotretinoin,[15] an oral retinoid. Accutane (Roche) was the first isotretinoin available for treatment of cystic, scarring acne, followed by generic versions Amnesteem (Genpharm), Claravis (Barr), and Sotret (Renbaxy). In mid 2009, Roche stopped production of Accutane, since cost-conscious users were turning to the generic versions. Isotretinoin shrinks sebaceous glands and reduces sebum secretion. This medication can be quite effective in clearing acne, but there are potential side effects, including extremely severe and deforming birth defects, depression and mood changes with possible suicidal attempts, bony changes, eye changes, pancreatitis, inflammatory bowel disease, hearing impairment, liver toxicity, visual impairment, hair loss, and others. Facial skin becomes very dry during treatment with isotretinoin.

Isotretinoin is contraindicated in females of childbearing potential unless they have severe, disfiguring, nodular acne that is recalcitrant to standard therapies. Females in childbearing years must have two negative pregnancy tests prior to starting medication. They must commit to using two forms of contraceptives simultaneously, and contraception must be used for at least one month prior to therapy and for one month following discontinuation of therapy. Treatment is usually for 15 to 20 weeks. If a second course of therapy is necessary, at least 8 weeks should lapse after completion of the first course. Prescriptions can be filled only on a monthly basis and only after negative pregnancy testing and contraception counseling each month. Consultation and follow-up with a dermatologist is required to understand potential problems and for monitoring during treatment with isotretinoin[16] or any other medication.

I have tiny bumps all over my forehead that won't go away. I use the best products—a night cream that's very expensive and a day cream from the same line. What is wrong?

—Kay, age 32

Avoid heavy creams and ointments on your face. These can clog pores and make acne worse. If you have dry skin and need to use a moisturizer, use a noncomedogenic moisturizer such as Purpose, Moisturel, or Nutraderm after washing your face. Some hair products, including conditioners, can cause acne lesions on the forehead or on the back and shoulders where hair hangs.

I keep breaking out with acne and the spots turn dark and won't go away. What can I do?

—Shala, age 28

Hispanics, Asians, and African Americans have increased risk for developing dark patches (post-inflammatory hyperpigmentation) as inflammatory acne lesions fade. The dark patches can last for months, so it is important to start treatment of inflammatory acne early to reduce the incidence of such hyperpigmentation. Topical tretinoin (Retin-A[17]), if not irritating to skin, can be helpful in treating the post-inflammatory hyperpigmentation of inflammatory acne. Azelaic acid (Azelex Cream[18]) and tazarotene (Tazorac[19]) can also be helpful.

Bleaching creams containing hydroquinone, such as Tri-Luma (prescription), can be helpful in lightening the dark spots. But most important is treating acne so that new spots do not arise.

I just turned 32 and my face is broken out with acne just like when I was a teenager. The dermatologist prescribed the same gels that I used in my teens. Aren't there any new treatments for acne?

—Carol Ann, age 32

Acne usually, but not always, begins to clear after the teen years, but many people find that they have another episode of adult acne in their 20s or 30s and sometimes even in their 40s. Many of the same prescription creams and gels used for many years are still good treatments for acne. New strengths are available in many of the prescription products. For example, Differin 0.1 percent gel now is also available in a 0.3 percent gel strength. The list of new products, however, grows each day. Topical dapsone 5 percent gel, an entirely new type of acne treatment, was added in November 2008. Oral dapsone has been used for years for treatment of a skin condition called dermatitis hepetiformis, but has only recently become available for treatment of acne. It appears to be effective in treating inflammatory acne, the type of acne with very red and angry bumps.

New techniques are also available for treating acne. Treatment of acne with certain (diode) lasers can be helpful. The Smoothbeam laser was the first FDA-approved diode laser for acne treatment. This laser targets the overactive, sebum-producing sebaceous glands. Exposure of skin to low-intensity blue light (Blu Light therapy) may also be helpful. The light is thought to destroy the bacteria associated with acne.

New "combination" treatments for acne are also available, where two or more techniques are used to attack different components of acne. The FDA has approved a combination therapy that involves pulsed light plus heat to treat mild to moderate acne. Pulses of green-yellow light plus heat destroy bacteria associated with acne and shrink overactive sebaceous glands associated with acne. Photopneumatic therapy for acne is another combination therapy that appears promising. Photopneumatic therapy combines IPL plus gentle suction that lifts the sebaceous glands closer to the skin's surface for removal of the sebaceous gland contents. Broadband blue light (400nm) is then used to kill bacteria associated with acne, and infrared (1,200nm) light is used to reduce inflammation.

New combination medications are also available. Instead of applying an acne medication in the morning and another at night, many medications have been combined to result in one cream or gel to be applied once a day. New low-dose antibiotics are also available for once a day treatment.

Chemical peels and microdermabrasion can also be helpful in treating acne. The peels remove dead skin and unclog pores. Microdermabrasion polishes the skin surface, exfoliating skin and unclogging pores.

Each case of acne is different. If you have acne, be sure to see your dermatologist to find out what treatment will be best for you.

I have mild acne. My dermatologist prescribed some acne gels, but my insurance won't pay for my purchase of the products, and they are just too expensive. I get acne only around the time of my period, and then it's just a few bumps. Isn't there anything over the counter that I can use?

—Carmella, age 28

There are many over-the-counter products available for treating mild acne. The most effective products contain benzoyl peroxide, salicylic acid, or sulfur and resourcinol. Such products are available in a wide range of washes, creams, and gels.

Benzoyl peroxide products kill the bacteria, *Propionibacterium acnes*, associated with acne. These products are available in strengths ranging from 2.5 percent to 10 percent. Be careful to rinse well after using a benzoyl peroxide wash. The products contain peroxide, which can bleach clothing, bed sheets, or towels. Because of the bleaching potential, when benzoyl peroxide washes are used on chest, back, and upper arms, be sure to rinse well. Confine benzoyl peroxide creams and gels to the face, and be sure to sleep on a white pillowcase that won't be harmed by bleaching. Benzoyl peroxide products can be drying. Some people are especially sensitive to benzoyl peroxide products. Decrease use if skin is dry, or stop using the product if there is any burning or stinging of skin. Benzoyl peroxide products can also make your skin more sensitive to ultraviolet light. Be sure to protect from the sun.

Salicylic acid products help prevent pores from clogging. This clogging occurs when cells inside the hair follicle shed. Salicylic acid products usually range in strength from 0.5 percent to 2 percent salicylic acid. These products can be helpful in treating blackheads and whiteheads. Salicylic acid products may also be somewhat drying. Alternate use of salicylic acid products with a mild, unscented soap and a moisturizer if dryness occurs, or discontinue use if skin irritation occurs.

Like salicylic acid products, sulfur-based products remove dead skin and excess oil. These products can be helpful in treating small blackheads and whiteheads. The sulfur-based products also have an antibacterial effect.

Be consistent with use of the products that you use. You will see some results in four to six weeks, but true evaluation of how much you will respond to an acne medication will take two or three months. Be sure to see a dermatologist if your acne does not clear or if your skin becomes irritated.

My dermatologist prescribed medicine that cleared my acne, but now I have bad purple scars on my cheeks and chin. I'm so upset. Will I be scarred for life? What can I do?

—Norma Jean, age 25

As acne cysts resolve, a purple-red color is left behind. The purple color will gradually fade. This may take several months, but you'll see progress every month. Once the purple color fades, you may not notice the underlying scars. If, however, you do have noticeable scars, there are procedures that can be helpful. These procedures include microdermabrasion, chemical peels, and laser therapy. See your dermatologist or plastic surgeon for discussion of these techniques.

I'm getting married in a week, and this red bump has appeared right on the tip of my nose. My wedding pictures are going to be ruined! Is there anything that I can do?

—Cynthia, age 22

Oral antibiotics can be helpful as well as topical treatment, but these take several weeks to clear acne lesions. Another option is injection, by your dermatologist, of a small amount of steroid into the new acne bump. This can usually help an acne cyst resolve in several days to a week. See your dermatologist for the best treatment in view of your situation.

One thing NOT to do is to try to self-treat from your local cosmetics counter. Remember Mary, at the beginning of this book, who bought a whole line of products right before her wedding, and her face became very irritated. A week before your wedding is not the time to squeeze or stick the bump or otherwise experiment in trying to get rid of it yourself. See your dermatologist to make sure your approach is the right one to best ensure that your walk down the aisle will be as glorious as it should be.

ROSACEA (RED FACE)

My face is always pink, and sometimes becomes very red, especially if I've been in the sun or if I've been exercising. I've looked on the Internet, and I think I have rosacea. What can I do?

—Joan, age 42

Rosacea is a common problem, especially in fair-skinned men and women. There is frequent flushing of the face, and the flushing seems to last a long time. Tiny little blood vessels (telangectasia) may develop on the cheeks and sides of the nose, and there may be persistent pink bumps on the nose and cheeks.

My uncle always seemed to have a red face with lots of blood vessels. He had greasy-looking skin and a huge, bulbous nose. My mom told me that he had rosacea. Now I'm really worried because now I have rosacea. Am I going to develop a big nose, too?

—Ann Marie, age 38

"Rhinophyma" is an enlarged nose that can result from rosacea. There is a greater risk that this will happen in men with rosacea than in women with rosacea. If you have rosacea, see your dermatologist for treatment. Rhinophyma can be surgically treated, usually with good results.

I've heard that drinking wine causes rosacea. Somebody else said that eating spicy foods or drinking coffee causes it. What really causes rosacea?

—Candy, age 42

Scientists haven't yet discovered the cause of rosacea. One theory is that it is caused by an allergy to[20] microscopic mites found normally in facial pores. Another theory is that the blood vessels in facial skin don't contract as well as in earlier years, possibly due to years of sun damage or hormone changes. Few young people have rosacea. Rosacea typically develops in the late 30s or 40s.

Certain activities that cause the face to flush, such as exercising, eating spicy foods, drinking coffee or other beverages with caffeine, or drinking alcoholic beverages, can worsen rosacea. The face and nose can turn bright pink and sometimes feel hot and painful.

I have rosacea. I've heard that there is no cure for this. Is this true?
—Bobby, age 51

Rosacea is a chronic condition, but treatment can help. If you have rosacea, your doctor may prescribe creams, gels, or lotions containing azelaic acid (Finacea)[25] or metronidozole (Metrogel [21], Metrocream,[22] MetroLotion, or [23] Noritate Cream[24]). These can be helpful in diminishing facial redness.

Oral tetracycline can be useful in severe cases. Cosmetic procedures such as laser treatment or IPL treatment can help get rid of little blood vessels (telangectasia) on the face.

Ocular rosacea (conjunctivitis and blepharitis) can also exist, and persons with rosacea and itchy eyes should be examined by an ophthalmologist. The National Rosacea Society Web site at www.rosacea.org gives helpful information on rosacea.

If you have rosacea, avoid products that can irritate, such as topical tretinoin[26] or alpha-hydroxy products. Use a non-scented cleanser such as Purpose Soap or Cetaphil Soap for washing your face. Use sunscreens with both UVA and UVB protection.[27] Sun exposure can cause rosacea to flare. If a moisturizer is necessary for dry skin, be sure to use an unscented product.[28] See your dermatologist for further treatment with prescription products as necessary.

MELASMA (BROWN PATCHES)

It started when I was pregnant with my first baby. I started getting these dark patches on my cheeks—then I got them on my forehead and chin. I know I wasn't being faithful with my sunscreen at the time, but I had never had a problem like this before, even when I didn't wear sunscreen all the time!
—Monica, age 29

Dark patches on sun-exposed areas of the skin, such as the face, hands, arms, and the V of the neck, can result from sun exposure, especially in a pregnant woman or one taking birth control pills or estrogen replacement. This condition is called "melasma." An old term for dark patches on the face during pregnancy is "the mask of pregnancy."

Some people appear to be more susceptible to melasma than others. For example, those of Latin or Asian descent seem to be especially susceptible.

Protection from the sun is the best protection against melasma. If the condition is already present, your dermatologist can prescribe creams with bleaching agents such as "hydroquinone"[29] to lighten the dark patches. Most bleaching creams work slowly, and the dark patches may not entirely resolve. Be sure to test the cream on your inner arm before applying it to your face to make certain there is no irritation. If the cream should irritate your face, stop using it immediately. Products that irritate your skin can cause it to turn darker, and that's not what you want.

Some skin bleaching preparations with low concentration (2 percent or less) of bleaching agent can be obtained over the counter. It is important, however, to see your dermatologist for accurate diagnosis of your condition. There are other causes of dark spots on the face.

If you are using a bleaching cream with hydroquinone, avoid using acne products containing benzoyl peroxide or other products containing benzoyl peroxide or hydrogen peroxide, since dark staining of skin can result from using these ingredients at the same time.

Dark-skinned people must be especially careful when using bleaching agents containing hydroquinone. They are especially susceptible to "pseudo-ochronosis," a rare complication of using bleaching agents containing hydroquinone for prolonged periods. In this condition, permanent patches of gray or blue-black can appear on the skin.

Alpha hydroxy acids and tretinoin products such as Retin-A[30] and Renova[31] can also be helpful in lightening skin. These can be used along with a hydroquinone bleaching product if there is no irritation. Azelaic acid (Azelex[32]), a topical medication used to treat acne, can also lighten skin.

LARGE PORES

The pores on my face are so large. When I wear makeup it clogs in the pores. I'm so self-conscious about this. Is there anything that I can do to reduce my pore size? And what do I do to clean my pores?

—Alicia, age 38

Your pore size is genetically determined. You cannot change the size of your pores, but you can do things to minimize their appearance. Oily skin makes pores look larger. To reduce skin oiliness, avoid creams and lotions on the face, use an over-the-counter facial wash containing salicylic acid,[33] and rinse well. Skin will feel tighter and pore appearance will be minimized. Avoid overuse of such facial washes to prevent excessive dryness.

Retinoids such as Retin-A[34] (tretinoin gel) can also minimize the appearance of pore size but can cause dryness. See your dermatologist to determine the best treatment for your skin.

I have one large pore on my cheek. Can this be removed?

—Brenda, age 32

Some people have a single large pore. A large pore can be excised, but there will be a scar.

CHAPTER 19

THOSE AWFUL WARTS!

My child has warts all over her fingers, on her elbows, and on her knees. Where did she get these, and what can I do?

—*Clarissa, age 24*

Warts are caused by a papilloma virus that gets inside skin cells and makes the cells grow into a wart. Warts are often hard to eliminate. They are usually treated by freezing them with liquid nitrogen, burning them by electrodessication, or applying chemicals such as salicylic acid.

"Almost gone" isn't good enough when treating a wart. The wart must be treated until it is totally gone. If any of the wart is left, it can grow right back into a big wart again. It is important to follow up with a dermatologist as long as any part of a wart remains.

I have warts on the bottom of my feet that hurt and won't go away. What can I do?

—*David, age 42*

Many warts, especially thick plantar warts on the feet, are persistent and require many treatments to remove them. The skin on the bottom of feet is thick, and the wart virus can get deep into the skin and make itself quite at home. Getting rid of these warts may involve surgical paring and liquid nitrogen treatment every two or three weeks for several months, or even much longer.

If you have patience and time, you can try treating these warts at home with liquid salicylic acid preparations such as Wart-Off[1] (17 percent salicylic acid) or Clear Away Liquid Wart Remover System[2] (17 percent salicylic acid).

For plantar warts, you will probably need stronger preparations of salicylic acid, such as Clear Away One Step Wart Remover[3] (40 percent salicylic acid in a medicated disc with a cover-up pad) or salicylic acid plasters (available over the counter in the drugstore). File the wart down every two or three days with a pumice stone or metal fingernail file. Cut the salicylic acid plaster to the size of the wart, apply, and add bandage tape to hold the plaster in place (or apply the liquid form of salicylic acid and let dry). The salicylic acid will soften the wart so that you can file it down more easily in a couple of days. After filing down a wart, always wipe the area with alcohol so that you don't spread the wart somewhere else from the debris. Clean the pumice stone or metal fingernail file with alcohol. Reapply the plasters for another two or three days and pare again. Continue to repeat this process until the wart resolves. This is a long-term process.

I have warts in my private area. They aren't bothering me. Can I just leave them alone and will they go away on their own eventually?

—*Betty, age 38*

It is important for genital warts to be treated. Some types of papilloma viruses that cause genital warts can predispose to development of cancer.[4] Females should have regular checkups with a gynecologist for detection and treatment of vaginal or cervical warts. Sexual partners should be treated for warts to avoid reinfection.

Condylox Gel[5] (podofilox) is available by prescription to apply to warts in the genital or rectal areas. Condylox slows down the growth of cells containing wart virus and is usually applied three times a week. The gel can cause irritation, pain, itching, and bleeding, so it is important to carefully follow the physician's instructions.

A newer type of treatment enhances the body's own natural immune response to fight the wart virus. When viruses or other invaders attack skin, the skin sends out signals to call in the body's immune cells to fight against the invaders. Aldara Cream[6] (imiquimod cream 5 percent) is applied to warts to boost the skin's natural signals (cytokines) in order to better fight the battle against the warts.

Other promising treatments for warts, such as photodynamic therapy, are in development today. See more about this in Chapter 29.

MOLLUSCUM CONTAGIOSUM

David, my four year old, has little red bumps all over his tummy and on his arms. His little two year old brother, Sam, also has some of these bumps on his back. They are both scratching and I think I see more little bumps coming on both of them. What can I do?

—*Corina, age 25*

Molluscum contagiosum[7] is caused by a pox virus. Tiny pink bumps appear with a tiny indentation in the center of the bump. On children, these often appear on the arms, legs, abdomen, and back. On adults they are often found on the abdomen and in the pubic area. Molluscum is transmitted by direct contact with an infected person. The bumps will eventually go away as the body develops resistance to the virus that causes molluscum, but this may take a long time, and the spots may spread in the meantime by scratching.

Adults should be treated. Small children should also be treated if there are not too many bumps and if the treatment is tolerated by the child without too much emotional distress.

The bumps can be treated by the physician by spraying them with liquid nitrogen (this stings and bleeding can occur), by surgically scraping (curettaging) them off (this stings), or by applying a medication such as Retin-A (tretinoin) to the bumps. The latter can be tried for small children who cannot tolerate the other procedures. Applying Retin-A is not as effective as spraying or scraping the molluscum, and irritation of surrounding skin may result from the Retin A.

It is likely that additional lesions will emerge before the problem is conquered. Clearing molluscum, therefore, may take several visits. Follow-up visits after the initial treatment are very important.

CHAPTER 20

BITES AND INFESTATIONS

BITES AND STINGS

*I reached back to scratch my back and when I scratched, this big hunk of skin
came away in my hand. I was horrified. When I looked in the mirror there was
this big round area that looked black and red, and I went to the emergency
room as fast as I could. The ER doctor told me that I had probably been bitten
by a brown house recluse spider, and that I needed to see a dermatologist and
maybe a surgeon. That was four months ago, and I'm finally healing after having surgery to remove some of the area and spending several days in the hospital
getting IV antibiotics. I didn't know there were such things, but I'll tell you
what. I look for spiders pretty carefully when I'm up in my attic going through
old clothes. That's where the doctor said I must have been bitten. Funny,
I didn't feel any bite or anything at the time. But I sure felt something later.*
                                                                   —Eleanor, age 31

Your body can react in different ways to bites or stings from insects
(mosquitos, fleas, fire ants, lice), arachnoids (mites, spiders), or other creatures. You may develop a small itchy bump ("papule") or a big pink welt
("wheal"). Depending upon the insect involved, there may be itching, burning,
or stinging at the site of the bite or sting. If healing does not occur or redness
increases, see your dermatologist. Infection may be present that will need to
be treated.

Some stings can be potentially life threatening in sensitized individuals.
In those allergic to bee stings, difficulty in breathing and even death can occur.
Those allergic to bee stings should carry an emergency kit with epinephrine in
a syringe for injection. Such individuals also need to go to the emergency room
right away if stung.

Spider bites[1], such as those of the brown recluse spider[2] sometimes found in
attics and other places around the home, can result in large areas of necrosis
(dead skin with non-healing ulcers) that need special treatment. Brown recluse
spiders are found most commonly in the South Central United States. The bite
of the female black widow spider[3] can cause severe muscle pain and cramps as

well as weakness, sweating, nausea and vomiting, difficulty breathing, and other symptoms. Serious systemic reactions can occur with spider bites. The black widow spider is found throughout the United States.

Those fuzzy-looking caterpillars aren't really soft and fuzzy. Contact with the hairs or spines of a caterpillar[4] (caterpillar "stings") can cause severe skin and systemic reactions. Wash your skin well if you come in contact with a caterpillar.

Bites from ticks of certain species can result in Lyme disease or Rocky Mountain Spotted Fever. See your physician for bites or stings or if your skin is irritated from contact with any kind of bug.

HEAD LICE

My child came home from school scratching her head like crazy. The school nurse said that she has head lice and needs to see a dermatologist. Now I'm itching too. Where did she get these, and what can I do?

—Marianna, age 28

Lice cause severe itching of the scalp. These tiny creatures[5] live on the surface of the skin and in clothing. There are several varieties of lice, each with its own preferences for parts of the body to inhabit.

The head louse lives on the scalp and glues its eggs, or "nits" to the hairs. These nits look like tiny, white, stuck-on "dots" on the hairs. Sometimes the lice themselves can be seen scurrying through the scalp. To treat head lice, apply Nix[6] or Rid[7] (both over the counter) to towel—dry hair and leave on 10 minutes before rinsing. Repeat one week later. Combing out the nits is very important to getting rid of scalp lice. A vinegar rinse (half water, half vinegar) will loosen the nits so that they can be combed out.[8]

Pubic lice live within the hairs of the pubic region. These are often referred to as "crab" lice. For treating lice within hairy areas such as the pubic region or the scalp, Nix Lice Control Spray[9] sprayed on the areas can be helpful.

Body lice live in the seams of clothing. To get rid of body lice, clothing must be washed in hot water and ironed. Treatment for body lice may also involve topical cream or lotion as described below for scabies treatment.

Some lice can be very hard to eradicate and can easily infect others if not eradicated. See a dermatologist for treatment.

SCABIES

My husband has been itching like crazy for the past week. He went to see the dermatologist today and was told that he has scabies. He says that the dermatologist told him that the children and I have to rub a cream all over us tonight because we might have it too. How did he get this?

—Michelle, age 41

Scabies[10] are tiny little mites that get *into* the skin and cause intense itching. They also lay eggs in the skin and pretty soon there can be hundreds of these microscopic creatures. Very itchy little red bumps appear as the skin protests. Sometimes tiny little burrows, appearing as short pink lines can be seen where mites have traveled under the skin. The "victim" scratches furiously because of severe itching, resulting in numerous scratch marks.

IMPORTANT: Dogs and cats can be infested with mites that can cause intense itching in humans. "Mange" in pets is caused by a tiny mite that causes your pet to scratch violently. If your dog or cat is scratching, and especially if you notice "dandruff" and patches of hair thinning on your pet, take your pet to the vet immediately for examination.

The mites like warm areas, and are very often found in fingerwebs, around the waistline, including in the belly button, and in the genital area. They can, however, live anywhere on the skin and are easily transferred to anyone who comes in contact, however casual, with the infested person.

To treat scabies, an antiscabies (prescription) cream or lotion such as Elimite[11] (permethrin 5 percent) Cream, Acticin[12] (permethrin 5 percent) Cream or Lindane Lotion (1 percent lindane) is applied from neck down all over the body. The cream or lotion is left on overnight, washed off the next morning, and the process is repeated one week later. For those pregnant and not allergic to sulfur, the dermatologist may prescribe a sulfur-based ointment to apply instead of the usual antiscabies cream or lotion.

Sheets on the bed, bedclothing, clothes worn recently, and towels used should be washed and ironed on the morning following treatment. Quilts or other bulky items that have been used recently should be stored for a few weeks in a large plastic bag with the top tied tightly. Scabies cannot live long away from its human host. They may, however, "camp out" on other family members who have not yet reacted to them, and therefore the entire family of a patient with scabies is usually also treated.

If you suspect that you may have scabies, see your dermatologist for a skin scraping (a small amount of skin is scraped onto a slide and examined under a microscope) to determine if you have scabies. Follow your physician's instructions carefully since most antiscabies creams and lotions are insecticides that can cause toxicity if not used properly.

CHAPTER 21

UNWANTED SPOTS AND GROWTHS

"AGE SPOTS"/SOLAR LENTIGINES

I knew that I was getting older when I looked at my hands and saw the "liver spots" coming. I used to tan, but now these spots are on the back of my hands and on my arms and are growing bigger and I'm getting more and more. Isn't there anything that I can do? I'm not ready to be old yet.

—Frances, age 51

Solar lentigines[1] are dark, flat spots (macules) that often look like large freckles on the backs of hands, on arms, and sometimes on the face, chest or upper back. These "age spots" or "sun spots" are caused by the sun and become more apparent as skin begins to age and no longer tans evenly.

Sun protection is of primary importance in preventing solar lentigines. Treatment is not necessary except for cosmetic purposes. Solar lentigines can be treated cosmetically with some success by your dermatologist using chemical peels, liquid nitrogen, pulsed light treatments, or other treatments.

Be sure to have a regular skin check-up by your dermatologist to make certain that what appears to be a solar lentigo is not a melanoma or other skin cancer. Lentigo maligna is a progression of a sun spot into melanoma. Lentigo maligna is usually very dark brown or black, sometimes mixed with lighter shades. It is very important that you see your dermatologist for a baseline examination of any dark spots on your skin and if any spots change.

SEBORRHEIC KERATOSES

My 83 year old father has these big, ugly, dark wart-like bumps all over his back. Now I'm starting to get them! They are horrible! What can I do about them?

—Judy, age 62

Seborrheic keratoses[2] are scaly brown or black raised spots (papules and plaques) on the trunk, especially between the breasts in women and on the back in men and women. They can look like moles, but their surface is usually rough, like warts. These "barnacles of life" begin to appear in the 30s or 40s and can be quite numerous. Sometimes they itch.

No one knows what causes these to develop, but in people with many seborrheic keratoses, it is likely that the tendency to develop them may have been inherited. There is no need to treat seborrheic keratoses unless they are itchy, irritated, or have changed, but it *is* important to be checked by a dermatologist to make sure that they are indeed seborrheic keratoses and not a skin cancer. Don't try to diagnose a skin growth by yourself!

If seborrheic keratoses itch, or you just want to get rid of them, your dermatologist can spray them with liquid nitrogen or scrape (curette) them off. When sprayed with liquid nitrogen, these growths will become crusty and usually fall off within two or three weeks.

Removing seborrheic keratoses that are not irritated is usually considered cosmetic and is therefore not covered by most insurance companies, meaning that you will have to pay "out of pocket." Be sure to see your dermatologist to examine any spot that itches, bleeds, or grows rapidly.

SKIN TAGS

I've got these little growths all around my neck and under my arms. I feel so embarrassed when I wear something with a low neckline and all of these growths are just hanging there. Can't these be taken off?

—Monica, age 35

A skin tag[3] is a small, flesh-colored or brown growth of skin that usually hangs from a small stalk of skin. Skin tags can be annoying and painful if caught in clothing or otherwise irritated. Some people have skin tags around the neck or in the axilla or groin. Most, if not all, insurance plans consider removal of non-irritated skin tags a cosmetic procedure and will not pay for the procedure. Ask your dermatologist how much removal of these tags will cost, since you will likely have to pay "out of pocket" if you choose to have them removed. The tendency to develop these tags is usually hereditary; there's nothing that you can do to prevent them.

NOTE: If you have a large number of skin tags, your primary care physician may want to arrange for you to have a colonoscopy. In some cases where there are numerous skin tags there may also be numerous polyps in the colon.

SCARS

I've got this scar on my leg where I fell on some glass. It's been a couple of months since I fell, but the scar is still raised and puffy. Should I be putting Vitamin E or something on the area to help it heal?

—Lana, age 28

Should you apply Vitamin E or one of the salicylic acid plasters (Mederma) to a healing site to try to diminish scarring? This is not necessary. Neither of these will do a better job of healing than nature itself and can sometimes cause irritation of skin.

Is there anything that you can do to minimize scarring after surgical excision? Avoid stretching of muscles under an excision site with sutures—no working those muscles on the machines at the gym while the sutures are still present. Let the skin heal without further trauma to the site. Gently clean away any crust on the excision site with hydrogen peroxide (diluted in tap water). Apply antibiotic ointment such as Bacitracin or Vaseline as directed. Follow wound care instructions carefully. Never scratch a scar. If it itches, your dermatologist can prescribe a steroid cream to reduce the itching.

Sometimes in the process of healing, a scar may become very large, or "hypertrophic." Sometimes it even overgrows the boundaries of the injury or excision site and becomes a "keloid" scar. Dark-skinned individuals appear more prone to formation of keloid scars. Hypertrophic or keloid scars can be injected with medications such as corticosteroids, 5-fluorouracil (5-FU), or a interferon. The doctor will usually inject such scars at 30 day intervals until the scar flattens. Scars can also be excised, but there is the risk that another, larger scar may result. Scientists are studying the mechanism of scar formation to develop better ways to reduce scarring.

STRETCH MARKS

I've got these stretch marks all over my abdomen, upper legs, and upper arms since I had my baby. Is there anything that I can do to get rid of them?

—Mary, age 32

Stretch marks ("striae") often occur in pregnant women, in adolescents undergoing a growth spurt, in obese persons, and in weight lifters. These scars may be bright pink at first, and quite distressing to the person developing them. The pink usually goes away with time, but the stretch marks remain.

If you have stretch marks, the most important thing to do is to treat your skin gently. Use a mild, unscented soap for bathing and an unscented moisturizer. Avoid any perfumed products. Laser treatment as well as tretinoin[4] cream and Vitamin E cream have been used to try to remove or improve the appearance of stretch marks, but none of these treatments have resulted in significant improvement.[5] Tretinoin cream and Vitamin E cream can cause irritation of skin.

Although there is no good treatment for stretch marks nor any way to prevent them at present, they will not be very noticeable once the pink does go away.

RASH

RASH

I've got an itchy rash all over. What should I do?

—Brenda, age 52

See a dermatologist. Don't try to diagnose the cause of a rash by yourself. There are a million and one different rashes. A "rash" may be caused by heat, by cold, by things that come in contact with and irritate skin, by a viral infection such as a cold, by medications, by stress, or by a wide variety of medical conditions. A rash may be mild and easily treatable, or may rarely signal a life-threatening disorder, such as certain bacterial infections.

There are clues that can help the dermatologist in trying to determine the cause of the rash. Sometimes the location of the skin changes can help determine the cause. Contact with earrings to which a person has become sensitized will result in redness and scale on the earlobes at the site of the earrings. Hypersensitivity to a ring will result in redness around the ring. In other cases, a history of a recent viral illness may give a clue. Recent starting of a new medicine can give a possible clue. Whether the rash itches or not, where it started before it spread, how it looked when it first started, and any associated symptoms also give clues. In some cases a biopsy may be necessary to try to determine the cause.

POISON IVY

I was out in my garden pulling up weeds last week and now I'm getting these blisters on my arms. I think I have poison ivy!

—Genevieve, age 38

The rash from coming in contact with poison ivy is a type of rash called a "contact dermatitis."

"Contact dermatitis" can occur from "irritation" of skin by a harsh substance or it can occur because of an "allergy" to a substance. If caused by "irritation," the rash happens soon after the irritating substance has touched the skin. You wash dishes and your hands become red and irritated. You put your hands in Clorox Bleach and they blister. These are examples of an "irritant contact dermatitis" and your doctor will advise you not to let your skin come in contact with such substances. A steroid cream will likely be prescribed for you to apply to the irritated areas.

If on the other hand the rash is caused by "allergy" to a substance that touches your skin, the rash may not erupt for several days to a week or more after you come in contact with the substance. Suppose you woke up this morning with an itchy rash on your legs. About a week ago you were in the woods hiking in shorts and walked through a field of poison ivy. You woke up with the rash this morning. But the hike was a week ago! Could poison ivy still be the cause of the breakout? Yes. This is an *allergic* contact reaction, where your skin has become sensitized to poison ivy and the reaction may be delayed (seven to ten days). Just because you have never reacted to poison ivy before does not mean that you don't have a poison ivy rash now. Skin sensitivity can change. Likewise, you may have used a product all of your life without problems, but suddenly your skin can become sensitized to the product.

Here's another scenario: You woke up this morning with a puffy, red face. Your eyelids are swollen. You itch. Several days ago your neighbor was burning poison ivy vines in his yard next door. The smoke drifted over into your yard while you were cutting some flowers. But you didn't get near the poison ivy. Could you have gotten poison ivy from the smoke? Yes. Contact with smoke particles from burning poison ivy or oak can result in an "airborne allergic contact dermatitis."

Your dog has run through a patch of poison ivy. If you pet him, can you get poison ivy? Yes, if he has gotten the oil from the poison ivy plant on his fur and you come in contact with it. Likewise, your garden gloves that pulled up the poison ivy can transmit the oil to your skin. It takes only a miniscule amount of oil from the plant to result in an allergic contact reaction. All of these reactions to poison ivy assume that you have been sensitized to (are allergic to) poison ivy.

Can you transfer poison ivy from one part of your body to another by scratching the rash? No. Not unless you still have the oil[1] on your skin. The fluid inside the poison ivy "blister" won't spread the rash. That's just your skin's reaction to the poison ivy. Remember, it's the plant *oil* that causes the rash. If you have taken a bath since you were exposed, you should have washed off the oil. But your garden clothes may still have oil on them if they have not yet been washed.

Antihistamines, such as Benadryl, taken *by mouth (oral)* can relieve some of the itching associated with poison ivy. Be careful since oral antihistamines can cause drowsiness. Lotions such as Calamine Lotion can be soothing, but avoid lotions and creams that contain antihistamines (Benadryl). Such products can sensitize skin, making the problem worse. If you have a severe case of poison ivy, your doctor may prescribe oral steroids and oral antihistamines.

Is there anything that you can do to prevent poison ivy? The best prevention, of course, is avoiding the poison ivy plant. Know what poison ivy, poison oak, and poison sumac look like, and avoid them! See http://www.poison-ivy.org for photographs of poison ivy and poison sumac.

If contact dermatitis is suspected but the cause cannot be determined, your dermatologist can perform a patch test on your skin to try to determine the cause. Remember, there can be many other reasons for a skin rash. See your dermatologist for diagnosis and treatment.

DRUG RASH

My doctor prescribed a new medicine for my blood pressure, and one week after starting it I broke out in this rash. Could I be allergic to the medicine?
—Eddie, age 47

A rash may be caused by foods or medicines taken by mouth. Flavorings, preservatives, antioxidants, spices, and dyes[2] are sometimes associated with rashes or other types of allergic reactions. Any medicine can potentially cause a drug rash. If you are allergic to a medicine, your reaction could be minor or deadly, depending upon your own, individual sensitivity to the medicine.

See your physician immediately if a rash develops while you are taking a medication or even after you have been off of it for a week or so. Remember that "medications" include non-prescription drugs such as aspirin, laxatives, and herbal remedies as well as prescription drugs.

HIVES

I woke up yesterday with this red, puffy rash all over and I was itching so badly that I had to go to the Emergency Room, where I got a shot that helped some, but I'm still itching like crazy. This is terrible! I ate some shrimp the night before the rash started. Could this be the cause?
—Rhonda, age 28

WHAT HAPPENS WHEN YOU HAVE A PATCH TEST

The doctor or doctor's assistant applies a series of patches on your back. Each patch contains a different substance that may be causing the rash. The patches are left on for several days, and then you return to the doctor's office to have the patches removed. If you react to the substance on one or more of the patches, the skin underneath the patch will be red and puffy. This test will help you learn some of the substances that can cause your skin to become irritated, so that you can avoid these substances.

A rash can have many different appearances. There may be lots of tiny pink bumps, there may be blisters, there may be a hundred different appearances. "Hives," or "urticaria" in dermatology language, is one type of "rash" that can happen with an allergic reaction.

With "hives," there are puffy, red, intensely itchy spots or areas ("wheals") that tend to appear and disappear. There are many different things that can cause hives, depending upon an individual's particular sensitivities (allergies). For example, one person may develop hives after eating shrimp, another after eating nuts, another after eating chocolate or fried foods, and another after drinking beer or wine. Still another may never develop hives after eating these foods. Another may have eaten a certain food all of his or her life, then suddenly develop an allergy to it. Certain medicines or viral illnesses can also cause hives in one person but not in another.

If you develop hives, your doctor will try to help you determine what is causing the problem. He or she may order some blood tests or allergy tests. If the cause can be determined, avoiding the cause should eliminate the problem. But often the cause cannot be determined, and the hives may eventually resolve. Oral (by mouth) antihistamines can give relief from itching. Your doctor may prescribe Allegra[3] (fexofenadine hydrochloride), Claritin[4] (loratadine), Zyrtec[5] (cetirizine hydrochloride), or other antihistamines. Oral benadryl (diphenhydramine hydrochloride), available over the counter, can be helpful. Remember that antihistamines can cause drowsiness. Never drive an automobile or operate heavy machinery when taking antihistamines that may make you sleepy.

If you have hives, it is important to avoid all substances potentially irritating to skin. Avoid perfumed products. Use a mild, unscented soap for bathing. Apply unscented moisturizer after bathing. If a particular food or food additive is suspected as the cause of the hives, your dermatologist may recommend a bland diet until the hives resolve. The food groups should then be added back one by one.

Hives can sometimes be long-lasting, and in some cases can be severe and life-threatening. If you develop hives and experience difficulty breathing, go to the emergency room immediately. Keep a diary of when the rash started, when it became worse. Record on a daily basis what time of day it is worse, and when it is better. Record on a daily basis what you have eaten, taken as medication, or applied to your skin. Include soaps or lotions used, cosmetics applied. Determining the cause of hives often requires such careful "detective work" and will be well worth the effort.

ECZEMA

I've had eczema all of my life. The smallest irritation to my skin and it becomes red and itchy. If I ever use any perfumed soap or lotions, I'm in real trouble with my skin. What's the best skin care for my type of skin?

—Amelia, age 29

Eczema is a chronic disorder characterized by scaling and redness on the arms, legs, hands, face, or all over the body. There appears to be a genetic component in susceptibility to eczema, although there can be sporadic cases without any family history. Atopic dermatitis is a form of eczema that usually begins in childhood. Itching can be severe. There can be flares of eczema, with quiet periods in between. Infection of skin with eczema can occur, causing flare-ups that can require treatment with oral antibiotics.

A mild soap[6] for gentle cleansing and a moisturizer[7] are important in daily care of skin prone to eczema. Anti-inflammatory agents such as topical steroids are useful for treatment of eczema. New treatments are also now available that block production and release of specific substances (cytokines) that cause the inflammation (redness) and itching associated with eczema. Tacrolimus[8] and pimecrolimus[9] are examples of these new topical, non-steroid therapies useful for mild to severe eczema.

Avoid scratching. Over-the-counter menthol products such as Sarna Lotion can be used topically to quell itching. Avoid perfumes and perfumed products. See your dermatologist for treatment and follow-up. For more information on eczema see the National Eczema Society Web site at www.eczema.org.

Read more about eczema in this book in Chapter 28.

PITYRIASIS ROSEA

I thought I had a ringworm on my neck a couple of weeks ago. It went away, but now I have a rash all over my chest and back and it's going down my arms. It doesn't itch, but it's spreading everywhere. What is happening to me?

—Carla, age 28

Pityriasis rosea is a rash that usually begins with a pink, scaly, oval "herald patch" that looks like a ringworm. This patch can occur on any part of the body. One or two weeks after the herald patch has appeared, small, pink, oval, scaling patches appear on the trunk. Occasionally these patches may itch, but for the most part they are asymptomatic. On the back, the small oval patches align themselves along the skin fold lines, in what is sometimes referred to as a "Christmas tree pattern."

The rash usually goes away within six to eight weeks. There is no known cause of the rash and no specific treatment. Use a mild, unscented soap for bathing, an unscented moisturizer after bathing, and Sarna Lotion for itching. As with any rash that persists, see a dermatologist for correct diagnosis.

CHAPTER 23

SKIN INFECTIONS

"RINGWORM" AND OTHER FUNGAL INFECTIONS

My son has pink, itchy circles on his arms and legs, and the doctor said that he has ringworm. Does this mean that he has a worm in his skin?

—Jesse, age 25

"Ringworm" is caused by a fungus. The "rash" of ringworm (or "tinea corporis") sometimes looks like pink, scaly circles. The fungus can infect skin, scalp, fingernails, feet, toenails, or any other part of the body.

Fungal infections on skin are usually treated with an antifungal cream and sometimes with oral (by mouth) medication. Prescription creams for treating fungal infections include Lamisil [1] (terbinafine hydrochloride), Nizoral [2] (ketoconazole), Loprox[3] (ciclopirox) (cream or lotion), Mentax[4] (butenafine hydrochloride), Naftin[5] (naftifine hydrochloride), or Oxistat[6](oxiconazole nitrate) (cream or lotion). These are usually applied twice a day to the fungal infection. Lotrimin[7] (clotrimazole) (cream, solution, or lotion), is available over the counter for applying twice a day.

It is important to see a dermatologist to diagnose what you may think is a fungal infection before you try to treat yourself with over-the-counter medications. Certain medical conditions such as diabetes, as well as living in a hot, humid climate, may predispose to fungal infection.

My dog has a red, scaly skin infection and I have what looks like ringworm. Could I have gotten this from my dog?

—Miranda, age 32

Dogs, cats, cows, horses, and other animals can have fungal infections as well as humans. *Microsporum canis* is the fungus that most often infects dogs and cats. This is often seen on the pet as a red, scaly area most commonly on ears, nose, tail, or paws, but can be found on any hair-bearing area. *Microsporum canis* can also be transmitted to humans.

If your pet has a skin condition, be sure to take it to the veterinarian for treatment, and see your dermatologist if you also have a rash. Your dermatologist can determine if a fungal infection is present by scraping a small amount of the affected skin onto a slide and examining it under a microscope.

THICK NAILS: FUNGAL INFECTION

My toenails are so ugly that I can't wear sandals in the summertime. The toenails on my two big toes are yellow and so thick that I have a terrible time trimming them. What can I do!

—Kristin, age 35

There are many causes of thick toenails or fingernails, but one of the most common causes is fungal infection. The nails often appear yellow-white as well as thickened. Applying Penlac Nail Lacquer[8] (ciclopirox) or Oxistat[9] (oxiconazole nitrate) lotion (prescription) can be helpful in reducing spread of toenail or fingernail fungus to other toenails or fingernails, but the nails can take a long time to clear, if at all—sometimes a year or more.

Antifungal pills are much more effective for treating fungal infections of the nails, but rarely there can be potentially serious side effects such as liver failure. Those that may be prescribed include Sporonox[10] (itraconazole) or Lamisil[11] (terbinafine hydrochloride tablets).[12] Because of potential side effects of antifungal pills, many people choose to apply the prescription lacquers or lotions. If you have thick nails, see your dermatologist to determine the cause.

DANDRUFF

My child is always scratching his scalp. He has this dandruff that is getting worse and worse.

—Melinda, age 24

"Dandruff" in young children often means fungal infection (tinea capitis). Fungal infection of the scalp and hair is common in children. The child should be examined by a dermatologist to determine if fungal infection is present.

Most "dandruff" in adults, on the other hand, is not fungal but instead is a condition called seborrheic dermatitis, discussed elsewhere in this chapter.

ATHLETE'S FOOT

I play a lot of tennis, and in the summertime I get a really bad rash between my toes. It itches and the skin starts peeling until it sometimes bleeds.

—Bruce, age 38

"Athlete's foot," or "tinea pedis" is a common fungal infection of the feet. There is often extensive peeling and cracking of skin between the toes, the soles of the feet are often red and scaly, and sometimes there are blisters in the foot arch. The rash can extend up the sides of the feet, giving the foot the appearance of wearing red, scaly "moccasins." Athlete's foot can be treated with antifungal creams such as Nizoral Cream applied twice a day. It's important to try to keep the feet cool and dry. Wearing sandals when possible will help. If the skin is not blistered and cracked, soaking feet in water with a little vinegar mixed in can help treat athlete's foot, but don't try this if the skin is broken.

JOCK ITCH

I keep getting this itchy red rash in my groin. I use antifungal powder, but it's still there. It seems worse in summer, but I also get it sometimes in winter.
—David, age 42

"Jock itch," or "tinea cruris," is a common fungal infection. This is a red, scaling rash in the groin with infection usually by yeast or fungi. Wearing loose undershorts to keep this area cool will help. Your doctor may prescribe an antifungal, anti-yeast cream such as Nizoral Cream, to apply twice a day.

SHINGLES

It started with stinging and burning on my abdomen. Then where this was happening, the skin turned bright pink. The pink began to spread around to my back, and big blisters began to develop. I felt like my skin was burned, it hurt so much. The pink kept spreading but stayed on only one side of my body—from the middle of my abdomen around to the middle of my back. I didn't think anything could hurt so much. Over the next three weeks I got more blisters, and then they began to pop and become crusty. Finally they went away, but two years later now and I still have shooting pains sometimes where the blisters were.
—Danielle, age 42

Having shingles[13] ("herpes zoster"), is a memorable event that no one would want to have. Danielle describes well what it is like to have shingles. The blisters ("bullae") and skin redness can appear anywhere, but will spread in a "dermatomal" distribution, that is, along one of the major nerve branches in skin. This "rash" could appear in a streak with blisters down the arms, down one side of the back or chest, or in any other streak along the affected nerve branch. The rash usually occurs on one side of the body or the other but does not normally cross the midline.

The official name of shingles, "herpes zoster" sounds as though it is caused by a herpes virus. And like "cold sores" and other herpes infections, shingles causes skin to sting and burn. But herpes zoster isn't caused by the herpes virus; it's actually caused by the "varicella zoster" virus—the same virus that causes chicken pox! But how can that be? Chicken pox is usually a childhood disease.

Yes, but once you have chicken-pox, the virus never goes away. Instead, it hides in the body in the sensory nerve roots ("ganglia"). Shingles is a reactivation of this virus. Reactivation can be due to stress, illness, or a number of other factors.

One of the unfortunate after-effects of shingles is painful "post-herpetic neuralgia," characterized by "shooting pains" in the skin that can continue long after the skin problems have resolved. There are effective oral antiviral medications that your doctor can prescribe when stinging and burning first start that will help reduce the incidence of future "post-herpetic neuralgia." These medications include Zovirax[14] (acyclovir), Famvir[15] (famciclovir), and Valtrex[16] (valacyclovir hydrochloride). See your physician if your skin begins to sting and burn or develop blisters.

"ID REACTION": A PROTEST BY YOUR SKIN

I had a really bad rash on my feet that my doctor said was a fungal infection. I thought I had the fungus on my arms and chest also because there was a rash all over those areas too. But my doctor did a test and said that the rash on my arms and chest wasn't a fungal infection, but was an "id reaction." What the heck is that?

—Edward, age 42

One of the strangest phenomena in skin is an "id reaction." This can happen if you have a really bad skin rash or reaction somewhere on the body. "In protest" to this skin reaction, your skin on a totally different part of the body can develop a rash. This is called an "id reaction."

For example, let's say that you have a bad fungal infection of the feet. Your skin may "protest" to such irritation by developing a rash on the arms. In such case the fungus hasn't spread to the arms. Your skin is simply "protesting." Treat the fungal infection of the feet and the rash on your arms goes away. This doesn't mean, of course, that you shouldn't have a dermatologist check to make sure that the rash on your arms isn't spreading of the fungus in your particular case.

No one knows what causes an "id reaction." It's probably a result of signals sent by the badly irritated area to other parts of the body through the blood stream to let the rest of the body know that there's a bad skin irritation somewhere on the body.

MRSA (METHICILLIN RESISTANT STAPHLOCOCCUS AUREUS)

I have a huge lump on my thigh. It is red and purple and hurts so much I can hardly walk. Someone said I'd better see my doctor because it might be MRSA. What is MRSA, and how can I get some relief?
—Robert, age 24

In the past, becoming infected with methicillin-resistant staphlococcus aureus was a risk for patients in the hospital. Now more and more people are becoming infected in their own communities. MRSA is resistant strain of the bacteria, staphylococcus aureus. The bacteria is even resistant to methicillin, a very strong antibiotic.

MRSA can spread from one infected area on skin to others, and in patients with suppressed immune systems, it can spread to any organ(s). Treatment choices are limited. Sometimes sulfa-based prescription medications can be used. Sometimes tetracycline antibiotics can be used. Your physician will rub any drainage from the irritated area with a cotton swab (long cotton Q-tip) and send the swab to the laboratory, where a culture will be done to (1) see what bacteria can be detected and to (2) determine what antibiotics are likely to effectively treat the infection.

MRSA is infectious and can spread from one infected person to another. It is very important to see a physician for treatment. Sometimes an infected sore can be lanced and drained. A prescription antibiotic will be necessary in clearing the problem.

I have a sore spot on my lip that keeps coming back. My lip starts tingling and burning before the sore appears. Then is lasts about three weeks before it goes away. It seems to come back when I am under stress or around the time of my menstrual period. I am told that this is a herpes infection. Can stress cause this?
—Sally, age 25

Herpes simplex is caused by a virus. One you have the virus, it stays with you, although you may not realize that it is still around. The skin or lip will begin to tingle, then sting and burn as the sore ("cold sore") appears. The virus is transmitted from person to person by contact with a herpes sore. After the sore goes away, the virus hangs around in a nerve. There are no symptoms until something makes the virus "reactivate" and a new sore appear, usually in the same spot as before. Stress, excess sunlight, illness, or other body stressors can reactivate the virus.

There are effective oral medications such as acyclovir (Zovirax), Famvir, and Valtrex that can be prescribed by your physician to abort or shorten attacks. Be sure to see your physician if you have a problem with recurrent herpes.

TINEA VERSICOLOR

I have this scaly rash on my upper back and upper chest. It is pink and scaly but there are also some patches that are lighter than my skin. It itches sometimes, and when my skin is tanned, you can really see the light spots. I live in the South where the summers are hot and humid, and the rash usually appears in the summer. I didn't have this when I lived in a colder climate. What is going on?

—Bryan, age 28

Tinea versicolor is caused by an overgrowth of a common yeast, Malassezia furfur, that lives in the pores of normal adults. The condition is more common in warm, humid climates but can also occur in colder climates. Overgrowth of the yeast can cause a scaling, sometimes itchy, rash on the neck, chest, shoulders, and upper back. Sometimes the rash can extend to other areas. The yeast causes skin to become pale in areas, so that as the skin tans, the lighter spots are seen in contrast to the tanned skin.

Your doctor can diagnose tinea versicolor by scraping the skin and examining the skin scrapings under the microscope. The yeast can be killed by applying selenium sulfide solution, ketaconazone cream, or pyrithione zinc. Oral anti-fungal medications, such as oral ketaconazone, can also be effective. See your physician for diagnosis and treatment. Once the yeast is killed, the skin will take some time, often a month or so, to return to its normal color.

CHAPTER 24

OTHER ANNOYING PROBLEMS

RASH UNDER BREASTS

I've got this rash under my breasts that won't go away. I've tried baby powder and all sorts of lotions and creams, but it just keeps getting worse. It's red and raw now, and I'm at my wits end about what to do.

—Roxanne, age 51

Intertrigo[1] is skin irritation in warm, moist areas of the body where skin rubs against skin, such as under the breasts, in the axilla, groin, buttock crease, or between fingers and toes. The rubbing of skin against skin causes irritation, and yeast or bacteria are quick to take advantage in this warm, moist environment, causing infection of the irritated skin.

Your physician may prescribe topical creams such as Nizoral[2] (ketoconazole 2 percent) Cream or Vytone Cream to treat infection by yeast or fungi, or may prescribe an antibiotic if there is infection by bacteria. Keep the area dry and as free from rubbing as possible. Lose weight if your thighs are so big that they rub together when you walk. Wear cool clothing in summer, and change underclothing often.

RECTAL ITCH

I've got this terrible itch in my rectum. I clean myself well, and even use a hair-dryer after wiping myself after a bowel movement to keep that area dry. I use cleaning wipes. I do everything I can to keep clean. And yet I itch like crazy. What can I do!

—Leonora, age 38

First, Leonora should stop such vigorous cleaning after bowel movements. Gentle wiping should suffice. Too-vigorous cleaning can irritate skin around the anus and set the stage for infection by yeast that live in the rectum. Diarrhea can often precipitate irritation around the anus.

Using scented (perfumed) or colored toilet paper can also irritate the area. If you have irritation or itching in your "private parts," use only white, unscented toilet paper. Avoid cleaning wipes, hairdryers to clean the area. Avoid contact with perfumed soap or lotion. Sitz baths (sitting in a tub of warm water) can help cleanse and soothe. See a dermatologist for diagnosis and treatment. Your doctor may prescribe a cream such as Vytone Cream or Nizoral Cream that soothes and provides protection against fungi and yeast.

EXCESSIVE SWEATING

I have to attend a lot of meetings where I have to shake hands. Whenever I get nervous I sweat, and my hands are always wet with sweat. I am so embarrassed. And that's not all. When I go to a party I sweat under my arms so much that I have big damp rings there. I'll do anything that it takes to get rid of this problem!
—Laurie, age 25

Excessive sweating, or "hyperhidrosis," is a real annoyance. No one wants to extend a sweaty hand in greeting or know that the back of one's shirt or blouse has become soaked during a stressful event. Sweating is a natural phenomenon, and it is much worse not to be able to sweat. But this is little consolation for those who suffer from excessive sweating.

What can you do? First, and most important, try to reduce your stress level. This is of course easier said than done, but it is the best bet in reducing excessive sweating. Wear loose-fitting clothes and avoid becoming overheated. Use an antiperspirant on the area of excessive sweating. Dry your skin before applying the antiperspirant.

Your physician may prescribe a topical medication containing aluminum chloride such as Drysol[3] (aluminum chloride 20%) or Xerac AC[4] (aluminum chloride 6.25%) to reduce sweating of hands and underarms. Botulinum toxin injections (Botox[5]) have also been used to reduce sweating. The toxin paralyzes nerves that stimulate sweat glands. Anticholinergic drugs can inhibit sweating, but are not often used because of side effects that include dry mouth, dry eyes, and potential loss of urinary bladder spincter control.

Some people claim that use of a technology called iontophoresis can inhibit sweating. Iontophoresis is supposed to affect ions in skin, which has to do with chemical reactions in skin. Not many physicians are convinced that this technology is very helpful to reduce sweating. In cases of severe sweating, nerves that affect sweating can be cut (sympathectomy) by a surgeon, but this procedure can't be reversed and may be associated with increased sweating on other areas of the body. Finally, the skin containing the sweat glands in the problem area (for example, in the armpits) can be excised and replaced by skin grafts.

The bottom line is that it is best to decrease stress levels, wear cool clothing, stay cool, and use unscented antiperspirants. Take along an extra shirt or blouse if you are nervous about standing in front of a group to give a speech and feel that you will sweat through your clothes beforehand. Ask your physician to consider prescribing a mild tranquilizer if necessary. When hot weather comes and you are outside on the tennis court you'll be glad that you didn't use drastic, irreversible means to stop sweating. If you need more than this, consider Botox injections to paralyze the sweat glands.

ITCHING

I can't sit still in a movie or in church because I'm constantly itching. I use the best products—expensive soaps and moisturizers, and take only medications that my doctor prescribes. What is causing me to itch so?

—Katia, age 44

Itching (pruritus) can be caused by many factors. Anything that irritates skin, such as perfumed moisturizers or harsh soaps can cause itching.

Dry skin can itch. Applying a moisturizer after bathing, especially in dry climates and in winter, will help treat dry skin.

Medications can cause itching. See your dermatologist to discuss whether any of your medications may be likely to cause itching.

Allergies, insect bites, itchy clothes, dark dyes in clothes, and many other things can cause itching.

Infestation with scabies or lice causes intense itching.

Use a mild unscented soap for bathing and an unscented moisturizer after bathing. Avoid bath powder or perfume and brightly colored or dark materials next to your skin. Over-the-counter Sarna Lotion can be helpful in giving temporary relief. You can cool Sarna Lotion in the refrigerator to enhance its soothing effect. Avoid topical anti-itch treatments containing benadryl since topical antihistamines can sensitize skin and itching can become worse.

Oral benadryl or other oral antihistamines can be helpful in relieving itching, but can cause drowsiness. Some oral antihistamines are more likely to cause drowsiness than others. Even those that are not supposed to make you drowsy could, however, have that effect. Avoid driving a car or operating heavy machinery while taking antihistamines that could potentially make you drowsy.

Certain medical conditions such as liver damage and Hodgkin's disease can cause itching. Be sure to see your physician for a checkup to determine if other tests need to be conducted.

HIDRADENITIS SUPPURATIVA

I've got these horrible, sore boils under my arms and on my inner thighs. Sometimes they fester and drain. They have been recurring since I was thirteen. I'm embarrassed and don't know what I can do about them.

—Sabatha, age 23

Recurrent boils or cysts under the arms and in the groin are often caused by a condition called hidradenitis suppurativa. This is a condition involving certain sweat glands, called "apocrine glands," which are found in these areas. Hidradenitis suppurativa is more often found in women, especially overweight women. It usually occurs between the ages of twenty and forty. Sabatha should see her physician for diagnosis and treatment. Her physician can prescribe an antibiotic for hidradenitis suppurativa. In severe cases, isotretinoin may be helpful. Surgical drainage by a physician may also be necessary on occasion.

LOSS OF SKIN COLOR (VITILIGO)

I have these white areas on the back of my hands and also on my arms. My mother has white spots on her back and face. We are dark-skinned, and the white areas are very noticeable. Did I inherit this from my mother? What can I do?

—Regina, age 32

Vitiligo is a skin disorder with loss of color in skin. White patches of skin may be evident on any area of the body. Often these patches tend to be symmetrical. They may occur, for example on both anterior lower legs, on the backs of both hands, on both upper eyelids, or on both upper arms. At other times there may be no symmetry.

The tendency to develop vitiligo is often inherited, but in some cases may arise spontaneously. The onset is usually around ages twenty or thirty and may or may not progress to larger and more numerous white patches.

Vitiligo is more noticeable on dark-skinned individuals. It is difficult to treat vitiligo, but phototherapy may be helpful in some cases. It is important to wear sunscreen on the white patches, since these skin areas will be more susceptible to sunburn. Most people with small patches of vitiligo find that makeup that covers well, such as Dermablend or Covermark, can give satisfactory cosmetic results.

If you have loss of skin color, see your dermatologist for treatment options.

DARK LINES AROUND LIPS

The borders of my lips have become darker. My friends think I line my lips with a dark color, but I don't. Why would my lips become dark like this?

—Latricia, age 29

Darkening of the "vermillion border" of the lips can be a normal occurrence without any reason or it can be caused by a number of different factors. Dark-skinned individual are more prone to dark lip borders than light-skinned individuals. Irritation from a lip liner or lipstick can cause darkening of the lips as the irritation resolves. Certain medications, such as minocycline, can also cause lip and gum darkening. Hormone changes or birth control pills can also cause lip darkening.

A disease of the adrenal glands, called "Addison's disease," can cause darkening of the vermillion border as well as skin. Skin tends to have a "bronze" color in Addison's disease, and there may be associated weight loss and fatigue. If your lips or skin suddenly become darker, be sure to see a physician to check for any underlying abnormalities.

PRICKLY HEAT (MILIARIA RUBRA)

I go to the gym every afternoon and work out for about an hour. When I sweat, my skin stings. I feel like someone is sticking tiny needles all over my body. Why does this happen? What can I do about this?

—Nancy, age 40

The flow of sweat from the sweat glands can be blocked in skin by humid climates, heavy clothing, stress, or exercise. The blockage can occur in different levels within skin. When the sweat is blocked in the upper skin layer, the epidermis, "prickly heat" can develop. Tiny red bumps appear on the upper chest, neck, or back. The bumps may be itchy or painful, and often feel like tiny pin pricks.

The best treatment for prickly heat is to stay cool. Since that is not always possible, some relief may be gained by soothing lotions that contain menthol, such as Sarna Lotion. Be sure to use an unscented soap for bathing. Prescription cortisone creams can be helpful. If prickly heat persists, see your doctor for treatment.

FACIAL REDNESS

Facial redness is often caused by rosacea. Other causes include irritation of skin by wind, weather, sun, or facial products. Some people inherit the tendency to have numerous small blood vessels under the skin, resulting in facial redness.

Treatment of the underlying condition is the most effective way to diminish facial redness. There are prescription medications for treating rosacea. There are over-the-counter and prescription medications for treating skin irritation. Numerous small blood vessels under the skin can be treated with laser or IPL.

The cosmeceutical industry has recognized that even with these treatments there is often a tendency of some people to have persistent facial redness. There are, therefore, new over-the-counter cosmeceuticals that the manufacturers claim will address this situation. For the most part, these are moisturizers in cream, lotion, or gel forms, containing various additives. The additives may be botanical ingredients that claim to relieve redness and restore natural skin color or they may be anti-inflammatory agents such as Aloe vera or green tea polyphenols. They may contain a small percentage (0.5 percent) of cortisone, or they may contain various "natural" ingredients purported by the manufacturer to relieve redness by "natural" means.

Do these antiredness products work? Most are basically moisturizers that help repair the skin barrier. Whether there is additional help from the additives depends upon the underlying skin condition and the additives. Every person's skin is different. One person's skin may be helped by a product; another person's skin may be irritated by the same product. If you try a redness-relief product and it helps, keep using it. If it irritates your skin, discontinue use immediately.

Here are the three most important steps in addressing facial redness. The first step is to repair any defects in the skin barrier. A mild soap for face washing and an unscented moisturizer will help. The second step is to treat any underlying disorder contributing to the redness, such as rosacea, seborrheic dermatitis, acne, or eczema. The third step is to see your dermatologist for diagnosis and treatment tailored to your underlying condition and *your* skin.

CHAPTER 25

CHRONIC SKIN PROBLEMS

PSORIASIS

*My aunt Bessie had psoriasis. I remember that she had this really bad rash all
over her stomach and back and arms and legs. Now I've got a rash on my
elbows and knees that looks like her rash. Am I getting psoriasis too?*

—Janice, age 38

Psoriasis[1] is a chronic skin disorder that can involve all areas of skin, especially the elbows, knees, lower back, and scalp. The cause of psoriasis is
not known, although there appear to be genetic and environmental factors
involved. If psoriasis has occurred in your family, then there is a greater likelihood that you may develop psoriasis.

The rash of psoriasis looks thick, red, and often has a silvery scale on top.
Stress often seems to worsen psoriasis. There is no cure, but there are treatments
that will be helpful. In ancient days people with psoriasis went bathing in the sea
and basked in the sun. These treatments are still useful today. Most often, treatment today includes creams and ointments containing corticosteroids, retinoids[2], or Vitamin D (Dovonex[3, 4] (calcipotriene), Vectical).

Oral medications, such as cyclosporine,[5] methotrexate, mycophenolate mofetil,[6] or oral retinoids (Soriatane[7]) may be necessary in severe cases.[8] There are
potential risks with the oral medications that should be discussed with your dermatologist. Such risks include anemia, immunosuppression, damage to liver or
kidneys, high blood pressure, and others. Monitoring by your dermatologist is
important to detect signs of these potential risks. The medications must be
avoided during pregnancy or nursing.

Tar baths and topical coal tar ointments can be helpful in treating psoriasis. Tar
shampoos are useful in controlling scalp psoriasis. Corticosteroid foam[9] can also be
used for psoriasis of scalp or other parts of the body. Scalp oils such as Derma-
Smoothe (contains peanut oil), are helpful in removing scale from the scalp.

Exposure to ultraviolet light is effective for treating psoriasis. Some dermatology offices have "UV Light Boxes" where a patient with psoriasis can receive
UVB exposure to skin. Such therapy three times a week can result in dramatic

improvement. Coating the skin with a prescription tar preparation before exposure to UVB is also effective.[10] If there is no UV Light Box available, a little time
in the sun (but not enough to cause sunburn) will improve psoriasis.

PUVA (psoralin + ultraviolet A) treatment is helpful in treating psoriasis as well
as a number of other skin disorders. PUVA involves taking a medicine called "psoralin," followed by exposure of skin to UVA radiation. Psoralins are found naturally
in plants such as celery, and sensitize skin to ultraviolet light. This sensitization kills
cells in skin that play a role in psoriasis.[11] Potential side effects of PUVA therapy
include nausea, headache, fatigue, burning and itching. There is also an increased
risk of skin cancer with long-term treatment. "Narrow band" UVB or UVA treatment, which utilizes specific wave lengths of light to which psoriasis is most respon-
sive, can be more powerful than the traditional "broad band" UVB or UVA therapy.

Exciting, new treatments for psoriasis have emerged. New "immunotherapies"
block specific substances (cytokines) involved in psoriasis. In many cases this results
in dramatic clearing of psoriasis. See Chapter 31 for further discussion of the new
immunotherapies. For more information about psoriasis, see the National Psoriasis
Foundation Web site at www.psoriasis.org/.

SWOLLEN LEGS AND IRRITATED SKIN

*My grandmother has a terrible time with her legs. They are so swollen and the
skin is stretched so tight that it is red and weepy all the time. What is causing
this, and what can we do to help her?*

—Sandra, age 38

Poor circulation[12] results in poor return of blood from the legs back to the
heart. This results in edema, or swelling of legs. Elevating the legs can usually
reduce some of the leg swelling. Stretching of skin from swelling of the legs contributes to "venous stasis dermatitis," with rash and weeping of skin. Typically
the dermatitis is located on the lower legs and ankles.

Venous stasis dermatitis is treated by leg elevation, support stockings to help
the blood return back to the heart, moisturizers to relieve dry skin, and mild steroid creams to treat inflammation. Occasionally the skin will become infected
and antibiotics will be necessary. Sandra should take her grandmother to a
dermatologist for treatment of her skin and to her primary care physician for
management of the underlying circulation problem.

LICHEN SIMPLEX CHRONICUS

*There is a large spot on my right ankle that itches all the time. I try to keep
from scratching, but I can't. It itches too much. When I scratch, it feels so good.
Why won't this spot go away?*

—Bruce, age 42

Lichen simplex chronicus is a patch of skin that is chronically scratched. If the scratching stops, the patch will go away. But it itches, and it feels so good to scratch it. Sometimes people don't even realize that they are scratching—the scratching and rubbing have become a habit.

The initial problem is something that irritates skin. This may be a perfumed product, a medication that makes the skin itch, dry skin, a mosquito bite, poison ivy, or any other skin irritants. The irritation causes the skin to itch. Scratching temporarily relieves the itching, but the skin "defends" itself by becoming thicker, and develops more nerve endings. This makes the skin even more itchy, and a vicious "itch-scratch" cycle ensues. Infection from the scratching can complicate the problem.

The treatment is to stop scratching. Use only non-perfumed products—an unscented soap, an unscented moisturizer, and apply a menthol-containing lotion, such as Sarna Lotion, for relief of itching. In some cases an oral antihistamine may be necessary to further control itching, and an antibiotic may be prescribed to treat superimposed infection from scratching. Cortisone can be prescribed by your doctor to heal the skin and also give relief from itching.

Anxiety often precipitates or prolongs lichen simplex chronicus. Scratching an area of skin becomes a distraction from underlying stress, and the itch-scratch cycle continues. See a physician for treatment of lichen simplex chronicus and to help deal with stress that may be prolonging the problem.

CHAPTER 26

PROBLEMS IN AND AROUND THE MOUTH

COLD SORES

I can always tell when I'm getting a cold sore. My lip starts to sting and burn, and I know it's coming. It always seems to happen when I'm about to take an exam or go on a big date!

—Eloise, age 19

Cold sores or "fever blisters" are caused by the herpes simplex virus (Type I). The lip often begins to sting and burn where an outbreak is about to occur. A painful bump develops and forms blisters that will crust and finally resolve over two or three weeks.

Cold sores sting and burn and are unattractive. As if this isn't enough, it is very common for cold sores to continue to recur in the same place. Stress, sunburn, menstrual periods, and illnesses can precipitate outbreaks. Moreover, no one with a cold sore is very kissable. The virus can be transmitted to someone else who comes in contact with the fever blister.

There are medications that can shorten the course of a herpes outbreak if started when the stinging and burning is first felt. The medication is usually taken for five to seven days and reduces the painful outbreak to about a week in most cases. If you have a cold sore, see your physician for treatment with one of several antiviral medicines in pill form such as Zovirax[1] (acyclovir), Famvir[2] (famciclovir), or Valtrex[3] (valacyclovir hydrochloride). If you have frequent attacks of herpes, your physician may prescribe "maintenance therapy," which involves taking a small dose of antiviral medication each day.

CANKER SORES

I get these painful little ulcers on my gums or other areas in my mouth from time to time. They really hurt and last for a couple of weeks sometimes. I can't drink much of anything except soft drinks when I get them, and it hurts to eat. What can I do about this problem?

—*Randy, age 31*

Canker sores[5], or "apthous ulcers," in the mouth are very painful. Some people seem more prone to these than others. Sickness or stress may precipitate an outbreak. There are also some medical conditions that can be associated with canker sores. Over-the-counter

NOTE: The herpes virus can affect not only the lips but also the genital area, skin of the buttocks, or any other area of skin. Genital herpes[4] is usually caused by herpes simplex virus Type II. There are usually tiny blisters (vesicles) on pink skin, and the lesions usually sting and burn. As with cold sores, herpes simplex in any area can be spread to others through contact.

products are available or your dermatologist can prescribe gels or "swish and spit" medications to relieve discomfort. If you have recurrent problems with canker sores, see your physician for examination and treatment.

ANGULAR CHELITIS

I get these cracks in the corners of my mouth, and they become so sore that it's hard to smile or even eat. The corners of my mouth are so irritated that they even bleed sometimes. My lips feel dry, and I lick them to keep them moist, but the problem just gets worse. My husband says that he has heard that this is caused by drooling. I got mad at that. What's going on?

—*Cindy, age 59*

Cindy, you probably do drool—in your sleep if you aren't aware of it. That's OK. Many people do. But what is happening is a combination of things: (1) Licking your lips breaks down the skin and makes the skin irritated and more susceptible to infection, (2) Drooling puts yet more saliva onto sensitive skin and also brings the yeast found naturally in your mouth in contact with the irritated skin, (3) The yeast get into the irritated skin and create a yeast infection. It is likely that you have some little wrinkles in those cracks and this provides the perfect place for those yeast to grow.

What to do? See a dermatologist. He or she will likely prescribe a medication such as Nizoral Cream that will help kill the yeast and help clear the problem. It will be important for you not to lick your lips.

CHAPTER 27

SKIN CHANGES
IN PREGNANCY

I'm six months pregnant and growing more than my baby. Look at these red spots—there's one on the tip of my nose and another on my chest. And the mole on my upper leg is changing. What's happening?

—*Sue Ellen, age 28*

During pregnancy your body changes and you may grow new spots. They may be little or big, dark or flesh-colored or red, and may be perfectly benign or may be problematic. Skin growths and other skin changes during pregnancy are likely due to hormonal changes that come with pregnancy,[1] but it is best to have your moles and other growths checked to make certain that any changes are not worrisome.

Tiny new little blood vessels called telangectasia sometimes develop on the face, chest or other areas during pregnancy, and moles may change. Sun exposure without adequate protection with sunscreen and protective clothing may result in "melasma," or dark patches on skin. Skin as it stretches over the expanding abdomen may become dry and itchy. Skin conditions such as psoriasis or acne may actually improve—or may worsen—during pregnancy.

Rarely, a red, itchy rash called PUPPP (Pruritic Urticarial Papules and Plaques of Pregnancy) may develop over the abdomen and other areas during the last trimester of pregnancy. This is a type of hypersensitivity (allergic) reaction that will require treatment and careful monitoring by a dermatologist and obstetrician and usually resolves after the baby is born. Another intensely itchy rash that rarely occurs during pregnancy is herpes gestationis. In this condition there are large blisters on reddened skin. Despite the name, "herpes gestationis," this condition is not caused by the herpes virus. Like PUPPP, herpes gestationis is a hypersensitivity reaction during pregnancy and will require treatment by a dermatologist and obstetrician.

Skin during pregnancy requires the same good care that you should always give your skin: (1) a mild, unscented soap, (2) an unscented moisturizer if your skin is dry, and (3) sunscreen. For itching, try applying Sarna Lotion (contains menthol). Avoid topical antihistamines such as Caladryl.

MELANOMA AND PREGNANCY

I had a melanoma a year ago. The melanoma was excised and my dermatologist says that I should do fine now as long as I have regular skin check-ups. My husband and I would like to have a baby. Is there any risk that the melanoma will come back during pregnancy?

—Catherine, age 25

For many years there was concern of reactivation of melanoma with pregnancy. Because of this concern, many doctors recommended that a patient who had melanoma wait two or three years after treatment of the melanoma before becoming pregnant, since the risk of recurrence is greatest during the first two or three years after a melanoma has been treated. More recent studies tend to lean towards no more risk of reactivation of melanoma with pregnancy than if the person is not pregnant. In cases, however, where the melanoma has been deep enough such that risk of death from the melanoma is predicted to be greater than 10 percent, it is wise to wait three or four years before becoming pregnant.

Remember that there is always risk, however, that a melanoma, or any other skin cancer, can recur. The risk diminishes with thin melanomas and if wide excision has been performed to remove the melanoma. It is very important to have a regular skin check and to see your dermatologist if any mole changes in any way. Early detection and treatment of melanoma are of utmost importance during pregnancy as well as at other times.

If you have had a melanoma and want to consider pregnancy, discuss with your dermatologist the depth and prognosis of your melanoma and your risk with pregnancy. Follow your dermatologist's advice.

CHAPTER 28

COMMON PROBLEMS
IN CHILDREN

ACNE NEONATORUM

My baby is only a few days old and it looks like he already has acne! There are these little bumps on his cheeks and they look exactly like the acne that I had as a teenager. What's going on?

—Donna, age 24

S ome babies are born with what appears to be acne on their cheeks. This is called acne neonatorum[1] and is due to exposure in the womb to the mother's hormones. The acne will resolve within the first couple of months.

Donna should have her baby examined by a pediatrician or dermatologist to confirm the diagnosis and to make certain that the condition resolves.

STRAWBERRY HEMANGIOMA

My baby has a pink area on the back of her neck that looks like someone pinched her. And on her lower back is a bright red spot about the size of a strawberry. What should I do about these to make them go away?

—Wilberta, age 25

A strawberry hemangioma[2] is a collection of blood vessels that form a pink or red patch or a raised nodule on a baby's skin. There are different types depending upon the types and depth of blood vessels involved. Most of these birthmarks resolve by the time a child is eight or nine years old. There are a few types, however, that do not resolve.

A "port wine stain," for example, is a reddish-purple patch that can continue to grow, may bleed, and can be associated with underlying problems, especially if on the face. If your child has a birthmark of any kind, show it to your pediatrician or dermatologist to determine the kind of birthmark and whether any treatment is necessary.

If a hemangioma is large and involves the eye, nose, or other vital areas, oral steroids may be prescribed to help shrink the hemangioma. Laser treatment can also be helpful in resolving small, persistent hemangiomas. If your child's doctor says that your child's hemangioma is likely to go away on its own, however, give it time before being aggressive in trying to get rid of it.

MONGOLIAN SPOTS

My baby was born with big brown/blue patches on his back and rear end. Is this something to worry about?

—*Takesha, age 23*

Mongolian spots[3] are bluish patches on the buttocks or lower back of an infant. These spots are more common in dark-skinned babies and usually disappear within the first three or four years of life. They are caused by pigmentation deep in skin, and no treatment is necessary. Takesha will, of course, need to have her baby checked by a pediatrician or dermatologist to make sure of the diagnosis.

ECZEMA

My child is always scratching—on his arms, his legs, his stomach—everywhere. Nothing that I do helps. His skin stays red and raw, and really gets bad in wintertime. I'm at my wits end. What can I do?

—*Carol, age 24*

Eczema, or atopic dermatitis,[4] can be terribly uncomfortable for your child and can make you feel helpless in trying to do something for your child to help. In infants there is usually a very itchy rash over the elbows, on the cheeks, and on the legs. As the child grows older, the rash also appears behind the knees, on the tummy, and on the inner arms—in the areas that the child can now reach to scratch.

Eczema can make a child miserable with constant itching and the need to scratch. But this is a vicious cycle since scratching causes more itching, thickening of the skin, and sometimes infection, adding to the problem.

What can you do? First, make sure that you use an unscented soap for bathing your child. Dove or Cetaphil are good choices. Avoid antibacterial soaps. Avoid bubblebath or any scented bath oils in the tub. If you are putting a drop or two of baby oil in the bath water, switch to a little mineral oil—it's the same thing without the fragrance. Immediately after bathing—immediately after patting dry—rub on an unscented moisturizer such as Moisturel Lotion or Eucerin Lotion. This is the important daily routine.

Your child's doctor will also prescribe mild topical steroids as necessary to control flares or some of the new "biologics" such as Elidel (pimecrolimus) or Protopic (tacrolimus) for milder flares. Ask your doctor about side effects of the treatment prescribed. For example, long-term use of steroids, especially stronger steroids, can cause skin thinning. There are also potential side effects of Elidel or Protopic. These types of treatments are important in controlling eczema, but should be relied on for flares only, with mild soap and moisturizer the daily mainstay for control as much as possible.

Your baby has an increased risk of developing eczema if you or your spouse or a relative has had eczema. It is important to take your child to his or her doctor if sores develop from scratching.

"CRADLE CAP"

My baby has this thick scale all over her scalp. It looks terrible! Somebody told me that she has "cradle cap" and that I should put oil on it. What's going on? Is this something that she's going to have a problem with for the rest of her life?
—Anita, age 21

"Cradle cap," or "seborrheic dermatitis" of infants, is a common condition found in babies. There is greasy-looking, sometimes thick, scale stuck on the scalp. The scale doesn't come off very easily, and sometimes the scalp is pink and irritated. Apply vegetable or mineral oil to the baby's scalp to soften the scales. After the scales have softened, the scalp can be gently combed and washed with baby shampoo. Don't try to remove all of the scales at once—a little at a time will do. This condition usually resolves during the baby's first year of life. For more information about "cradle cap," see http://www.eczema-assn.org/seborrheic.html.

DIAPER RASH

My child has a diaper rash that just won't go away. I've tried diaper rash ointments and creams, but it just gets worse. There are big boils on her little bottom. What can I do?
—Amelia, age 24

Amelia's child, of course, needs to go to the pediatrician or dermatologist. She has a skin infection that will need to be treated by the physician.

Diaper rash[5] is usually caused by contact of a baby's skin with the ammonia found in urine, resulting in irritation and redness in the diaper area. But this area is also warm and moist, which predisposes the irritated area to secondary infection by bacteria or yeast.

Change your baby's diaper often. Cleanse the diaper area well, and apply baby lotions. If the skin is pink and irritated, apply diaper rash ointments (zinc oxide ointments or petrolatum). These ointments help protect skin from irritants in urine.

If a rash spreads or does not improve, take your baby to the doctor for further treatment.

IMPETIGO

My child has sores on his skin that are spreading. He scratched at a mosquito bite on his foot and the spot developed an oozing yellow crust. I thought it was probably infected, so I put some antibiotic ointment on it. But now he has other spots coming on his arms and legs, and he hasn't been around any more mosquitoes.

—Dana, age 25

It's hard not to scratch a mosquito bite, but doing so can result in infection. Over-the-counter hydrocortisone cream applied to the bite can give some relief as can a soothing menthol solution such as Sarna Lotion or if you are camping and in a bind for something to apply, apply a dab of menthol toothpaste to give some quick relief.

If a mosquito bite does become infected—turn red, become oozy—an over-the-counter antibiotic ointment will often work to eliminate the infection. In some cases, however, the infection is caused by certain bacteria that may require prescription ointments or oral medication (liquid or pill form).

Impetigo[6] is a contagious infection of the skin caused by streptococcal or staphylococcal bacteria. It is characterized by sores that do not heal, appear to spread, sometimes itch, and usually have yellow crusts. Over-the-counter antibiotics will not always work with certain bacteria that cause impetigo. Some strains of streptococci that cause impetigo can also cause damage to the kidneys. Take your baby to a dermatologist or pediatrician for antibiotic treatment if your child develops sores that do not heal.

RASH

My child has a rash. First she had a high fever. This went away and now she has a rash all over. What should I do?

—Rosemary, age 19

Roseola is a common childhood rash that can develop after a high fever has come and gone. Even though the symptoms of Rosemary's baby suggest roseola, it is important for Rosemary to take her child to the doctor to be checked. Measles, scarlet fever, chicken pox, bacterial or viral diseases, and many other infections can also cause a skin rash in children.

It is very important to have your child's rash evaluated by a physician, especially if it is associated with fever or other symptoms. Remember, there are many causes of a rash, some very serious.

PART V

THE FUTURE

CHAPTER 29

OH CRYSTAL BALL, WHAT IS THE FUTURE FOR US ALL?

Collaborations between company scientists and university scientists are resulting in exciting new products based upon "real science."

Pharmaceutical and cosmetic companies are always on the lookout for ways to address problems and satisfy consumers. A good product helps the consumer and produces profit for the company.

Not all products touted as new are really new. Because inventions in the laboratory take much time and money to turn into new products, scientists in cosmetic and health care companies often spend much time "reformulating" old products. This may indeed make creams smoother, less irritating, more appealing, and more effective as moisturizers, so that in this way the product is "new." But often what the company promotes as "new" isn't the reformulation, but some new ingredient with a

> • Many times a product touted as "new" is simply a reformulation of an old product.

catchy name or "in vogue" phrase claimed to be the breakthrough cure for wrinkles.

Consumers are becoming more educated and more skeptical of product claims. This creates greater incentive for companies to develop new products that really work in new ways. This requires new discoveries and the ability of the industry to turn such discoveries into products.

Most truly new discoveries occur within research laboratories of universities.

But scientists within university laboratories are often conducting "basic research"—that is, they are studying basic mechanisms—how the body works, what is necessary to keep the body working effectively, what goes wrong to cause diseases. Their quest is to understand and discover—not to develop a product.

Let's say that Sam, a scientist in a medical school research center, discovers a gene that makes new hair follicles develop on bald heads. That's a great discovery! But what can we do with that discovery to develop a product *now*? And how does an industry *know* about the discovery?

A savvy industry watches what is going on in the basic research laboratory. It surveys the scientific literature, attends scientific conferences, and acquaints itself with research that may be useful to the company.

> • Most truly new discoveries take place within basic research laboratories of universities.

In some cases the scientist may realize the potential of his or her research and contact an industry for development of a product.

Let's say that Company X spots Sam's research and sees an important connection between Sam's discovery and special expertise of the company's own "in-house" scientists.

For example, the company may have special expertise in developing creams that penetrate skin well, so that if a new ingredient was found that could stimulate hair follicles to grow, the ingredient could be effectively "delivered" into the scalp. The company may also have a collection of many substances that can be used for testing.

Why is the collection of many substances important? Gene therapy in general is not yet developed as a safe and effective tool. Therefore, we can't take the gene that Sam has discovered and put it into someone's scalp to grow hair.

But we don't need to do this. The gene would likely be present in the scalp but perhaps not in an active form. If the company can "screen" its "library" of substances to find one that "enhances" (stimulates) the gene that Sam has discovered, then the final effect can be the same: the screened ingredient could stimulate the important gene to be more active, producing new hair follicles.

This sounds very technical, but the bottom line is that industry needs the expertise of scientists, and scientists need the expertise of industry in order for a product to emerge.

So what happens next with Sam's discovery, now that a company has discovered his research? The company may propose a "sponsored research agreement" with Sam to conduct further specialized research to determine whether to go forward with development of a product. The company may send one of its own scientists to work with Sam on the project.

If the special research project yields information that is valuable to the company, the company may then take the project "in-house" to the company's own research facilities to apply the knowledge gained to perform further tests ("applied research") toward developing the product.

> • A savvy industry watches what goes on in basic research laboratories of universities to look for discoveries that can be turned into products.

The entire process of "translating" research "from research bench to product" may take years. There will be animal studies, followed by human studies, to make sure that the product is safe and works as planned. The process is very costly to industry and only the most promising results complete this process from start to finish to result in a product. This is the reason that

> • Turning basic research into a product can take many years and can be very expensive for a company.

companies often "reformulate" rather than develop truly new products.

When company scientists and academic scientists work together, however, a powerful synergy comes into play that can result in truly new products based on real scientific findings. For example, Shiseido, a Japanese cosmetic company has maintained a 20-year collaboration with the Massachusetts General Hospital/Harvard Cutaneous Biology Research Center in Boston. Shiseido's skin care lines, Qiora, The SkinCare, and Benefiance, were developed by Shiseido from observations that Shiseido gained from this collaboration.

Other companies with strong collaborations with academic institutions include Channel, L'Oreal, and Estee Lauder.

The future will bring more and more interactions between industry and academia as consumers demand products that work as advertisements claim. What can we expect?

> • When company scientists and academic scientists work together, a powerful synergy comes into play.

The next chapter will give a glimpse into research areas that will result in breakthroughs for skin care.

CHAPTER 30

HOT AREAS OF SCIENTIFIC RESEARCH THAT WILL CHANGE SKIN CARE

SKIN AGING, WRINKLES

I s your skin beginning to sag? Are you developing wrinkles? Discouraged by products that are claimed to help but don't? Hope is on the horizon.

Scientists that study the skin's "barrier function" are learning how skin creates its outer surface. They are discovering important new proteins that are assembled to develop an effective, intact skin surface that allows skin to maintain moisture and be protected from environmental stress. Exciting collaborations in progress between academic scientists and industry scientists will result in new creams and moisturizers to protect skin from dryness and cracking and to smooth and soothe skin for a younger, healthier appearance.

Scientists are also studying the interaction of skin cells with the substance (matrix) surrounding the cells. They are discovering signals that cells send and receive to carry on important functions in skin. These scientists are learning what signals stimulate cells (fibroblasts) deep in the dermis of skin to produce the proteoglycans, collagens, and elastins that provide

> Scientists are learning how cells send and receive signals to carry on important tasks within skin.

a youthful, firm foundation for skin. These studies will open the door for treatment of wrinkles down deep in skin where wrinkles originate.

"Angiogenesis" is the scientist's term for development of new blood vessels. "Anti-angiogenesis" means inhibiting growth of blood vessels. Scientists are discovering substances in skin that can stimulate development of new blood vessels or inhibit growth of blood vessels. Stimulating

> Scientists are learning how substances in skin can stimulate development of new blood vessels or inhibit growth of blood vessels.

development of new blood vessels in skin can enhance hair growth and lead to better wound healing. Inhibiting development of blood vessels has been shown to diminish skin wrinkling. Not only will the consumer benefit by new cosmetic treatments, but cancer patients also stand to benefit since inhibiting blood vessel growth of certain tumors can block further tumor growth.

PHOTOPROTECTION

Why can't we learn to control the cells that cause our skin to turn dark when we tan. Then we could just make cells give us a tan without having to expose our skin to the harmful rays of the sun.

—Sandra, age 40

Sunlight turns on certain genes that tell skin cells called melanocytes to produce pigment to tan the skin. Tanned skin gives some protection from the sun, but the process of tanning damages skin and increases the risk of skin cancer. Artificial tanning products that "stain skin" can give the appearance of a tan without having to damage skin from sun exposure, but unlike a natural tan, an artificial tan gives no protection to skin from the sun's rays. Scientists are now discovering ways to turn on the genes that the body uses to develop a natural tan. This research can result in a cream that won't just stain skin brown, but will cause skin to actually tan, giving protection from the sun without the need for harmful sun rays in order to develop the tan. The studies are in mice now and are not yet ready for humans, but results are promising.

SKIN TALK: "BIOLOGICS" AND "IMMUNOMODULATORS"

Scientists are not only discovering ways to improve skin tone, firmness, texture, and color by activating certain genes. Their research is also leading to new therapies for skin diseases.

"Skin talk," is the conversation that is passed from one cell to another so that skin functions can be carried out in a coordinated manner. Such "skin talk" happens largely through substances called "cytokines" that act as messages. These cytokines interact with other cytokines in "cascades" to result in different skin functions.

A beautiful symphony is composed of notes and chords played in a certain sequence and cadence, with emphasis and dimunition at appropriated times. Likewise, the many activities of skin result from cytokines and cytokine cascades in specific sequences and combinations, with emphasis and dimunition at appropriate times. A skin infection, for example, triggers a series of intricate and modulated cytokine interactions that call forth the body's immune cells to fight the infection. A skin cut results in a

> Scientists are learning how cells "talk" to one another through substances called "cytokines." This "conversation" helps cells coordinate their functions within skin.

series of interactions to bring cells and other substances to repair the wound. Sunlight sets off signals to stimulate melanocytes to make dark pigment (tan) to try to block further damaging sunlight.

"Skin talk" may be happy and normal in healthy states, but when skin is not healthy, this "talk" may be interrupted or inappropriately modulated (too weak or too strong), resulting in abnormal signals. Scientists have made exciting breakthroughs in developing the capability for understanding this language of skin. Scientists are not only making great strides in learning how to interpret "skin talk," but they are also learning how to target and block abnormal signals to restore normal skin.

Pharmaceutical companies are utilizing these discoveries to develop new "biologics" and "immunomodulators" to block undesirable cytokines to prevent unwanted skin changes and to stimulate desirable cytokines. Therapies are already available that "rev up" the immune system to fight an infection. Likewise, therapies are available that "calm down" immune cells so that transplantation of a heart or kidney can take place without rejection by the body. Examples of new "biologics" that treat psoriasis are discussed in the next chapter.

Finding the right notes, chords, and cadences to create the correct

---

"Skin Talk"

- New therapies determine what is "out of balance" and correct that balance.
- This may be done by destroying an unwanted substance (cytokine) with specific antibodies targeted to it, by specifically blocking its action, or by "revving up" immune cells.

"symphony" in skin is a challenge. For example, if immune cells are "revved up" too much, autoimmune conditions can result where the body's immune cells become too excited and begin attacking the body itself. If immune cells are calmed down too much, the body can't mount a defense against infection. Finding the right balance is just as important as finding the right cells or signals to manipulate.

CHAPTER 31

NEW BREAKTHROUGHS

PSORIASIS

I n ancient days, Egyptians with psoriasis were periodically buried up to their necks in warm desert sand to shrink the unattractive skin lesions associated with psoriasis. The raised, red, scaly plaques found all over the body in psoriasis would gradually diminish with such treatment, but the Egyptians could do little else while they waited for this improvement. There are few today with psoriasis who could afford the time necessary for such treatments. And who would not feel vulnerable buried up to one's neck in sand—especially with those camels walking around!

Others chose trips to the Dead Sea for bathing in the salt water to treat psoriasis. Some with psoriasis rubbed lard and other fats on the psoriatic lesions, improving the skin's appearance, but not its odor. The discovery was made that tar applied to psoriatic lesions was helpful in reducing the red, scaling plaques. Tar was combined with sunlight or with ultraviolet light for a stronger effect. But early tar preparations were very messy. More cosmetically appealing treatments came with the development of topical steroid creams. Such creams are still an effective way to treat mild psoriasis. Other types of creams, such as Vitamin D creams, were also developed.

Patients with widespread psoriasis tired of twice daily applications of creams to large areas of their body. A breakthrough for these patients came when physicians found that the anticancer drug Methotrexate[1] not only treated patients with arthritis but also those with psoriasis. Methotrexate has potential side effects, however, such as liver damage.

The ideal drug to treat an abnormal condition would be one that *specifically* targets and neutralizes a *specific* cytokine or specific invading cell and *specifically* restores a normal situation, *without* affecting other body systems.

Scientists have now identified cytokines produced in psoriasis that activate certain immune cells (T lymphocytes) to "rev them up." These "revved—up" T cells produce a cytokine called tumor necrosis alpha (TNF-a), which plays an important role in the development of the skin lesions of psoriasis. Scientists have now developed drugs that can specifically "neutralize" TNF-a with dramatic improvement of psoriatic skin.

Already in the marketplace are many new "biologic" therapies that specifically target and "neutralize" TNF-a or other cytokines in the TNF-a cascade. Each drug has a different mechanism of action to accomplish this. Alefacept,[2] a protein administered by IV infusion (intravenously), blocks the activity of TNF-a and improves both skin and joint manifestations of psoriatic

- Scientists have identified cytokines produced in psoriasis that "rev up" immune cells, causing skin lesions found in psoriasis.
- Discovery of this "skin talk" in psoriasis has resulted in the development of exciting new "immunomodulators" and "biologics" that block cytokines for treating psoriasis.

arthritis. Infliximab,[3] an antibody administered intravenously every four to eight weeks, "neutralizes" the action of TNF. Etanercept,[4] administered by injection twice a week, "mops" up TNF-a before it can act. Leflunomide,[5] an oral medication (taken by mouth) used to treat rheumatoid arthritis, has also been found effective in treatment of psoriasis. Leflunomide blocks multiplication[6] of activated T cells. Anakinra, administered daily by injection into the skin, is a new drug that blocks Interleukin-1 (IL-1), another cytokine that contributes to the skin lesions of psoriasis. Each of these drugs has potential side effects, some severe, that need to be discussed with a dermatologist when such treatment for psoriasis is sought.[7]

These drugs are having a dramatic impact on the treatment of psoriasis, as the search continues for specific drugs with fewer potential side effects. We will see more and more important breakthroughs in the treatment of psoriasis in the near future as scientists become more and more familiar with "skin talk."

Because these are relatively new products, there is the possibility that there are yet side effects to be discovered. In June 2009, Efalizumab (Raptiva), which blocks activation of T cells to treat psoriasis, was pulled from the U.S. market because of safety concerns after three patients receiving Raptiva developed progressive multifocal leukoencephalopathy (PML), an uncurable, almost always fatal, brain infection caused by a virus.

Laser therapy is also being investigated for treatment of localized plaques of psoriasis with promising results. The excimer laser is now FDA approved for treatment of small areas of psoriasis. The laser beam is focused only upon the psoriasis plaque, therefore normal skin is not affected. Side effects can include redness, blistering, and darkness of the treated skin, all of which usually gradually resolve after treatment. The treated areas usually require retreatment after about six months.

New topical creams to stimulate appropriate skin cell "turnover" are also available. In 2009, the FDA approved use of Vectical for treatment of mild to moderate psoriasis. Vectical (calcitriol) ointment contains an active form of Vitamin D.

ATOPIC DERMATITIS/ECZEMA

The skin can overrespond to certain factors, causing activation of T lymphocytes and resulting in eczema, or atopic dermatitis. Like overreactive soldiers rushing forward with guns firing, the T lymphocytes head for the skin, blasting away with cytokines called interleukins, causing skin redness, flaking and miserable itching.

> • Scientists have learned new ways to calm down immune cells to treat atopic dermatitis.

Scientists are learning how to calm down these T-lymphocytes and block production of interleukins that cause these skin problems. Drugs are already in use based on new discoveries in these areas.

Tacrolimus (Protopic[8]) is a non-steroid, topical (applied to the skin surface) ointment. The active ingredient binds to T-lymphocytes, "calming them down," preventing their production of cytokines that cause skin redness and itching. Pimecrolimus (Elidel[9]) is another non-steroid, topical cream that inhibits T lymphocyte activity by blocking production of cytokines.[10] Some skin burning and itching can occur with these topical medications, but the incidence of these side effects usually diminishes with improvement of the skin condition. There are other potential side effects that should be discussed with your physician before using these medications.[11]

SKIN CANCER

Whereas in psoriasis and atopic dermatitis immune cells such as T lymphocytes are "hyperalert" and need to be calmed down, there are other situations where "revving up" immune cells is desirable. If a T-lymphocyte attack could be directed specifically towards a skin cancer, for example, it is possible that the body could destroy many of the cancerous cells, sparing normal cells.

> • Scientists have discovered new ways to boost the immune system to fight skin cancers.

The body knows how to distinguish cancerous or otherwise damaged cells from normal cells, but often the body's response isn't enough to stop the cancer from spreading. If the body's immune response could be "boosted," a better response might result.

New treatments have now been developed that will boost the body's own immune system to fight skin cancer, warts, and other growths. Aldara (3M, imiquimod) is an "immune booster" that enhances production of cytokines to fight precancers, superficial skin cancers, and warts[12]. Other such immunomodulators with "immune cell boosting activity" are not far behind.

HAIR LOSS

Will there come a time when the round bald spot on the heads of men will disappear? When men won't have to do a comb-over across a balding scalp? When older women distressed over thinning hair will once again have thick, lustrous hair?

Yes. Drug companies are investing billions of dollars to find a way to restore youthful hair follicles. There's big money in it for the drug companies, and hope for those who despair over hair loss.

Is there anything in the marketplace that works to grow hair now? Propecia is an oral medication for men that will stimulate some hair to grow. This is not for women since it affects women's hormones adversely. Minoxidil may result in some peach fuzz or slight regrowth on the scalp, but little else. The optimum hair-growth treatment is yet to be developed, but scientists and pharmaceutical companies are getting very close.

Hair growth originates from hair follicles in skin. A continuous cycle of growth, rest, and renewal occurs in each hair follicle. Each hair follicle is on its own timetable—that is, some hair follicles are growing hairs, others are resting, others are shedding hairs.

Hair follicles need certain signals to start and maintain hair growth. First, there are signals within the scalp that tell a hair follicle to start growing a hair (anagen phase of hair growth). Second, there are signals that put the hair follicles in a "transition phase" (catagen phase). Third, there are signals that tell the hair follicle to rest (telogen phase of hair growth). Then the cycle starts over again with signals to grow a hair. Each hair is on its own cycle. At any one time, certain hairs on your head are in the anagen phase, others are in the catagen phase, and others are in the telogen phase. Imagine the complexity of "skin talk" going on in your own scalp!

When follicles finally "give out" in later years of life, they shrink (become "miniaturized") and stop producing hair. Scientists are studying how to "rejuvenate" these hair follicles. The key is in understanding the genes important to the development of hair follicles and in signals that maintain hair growth. Such genes and signals have been identified, and scientists are studying ways to magnify the "right" signals and block the "wrong" signals to regain and maintain the normal cycle of hair growth.

Scientists with pharmaceutical companies are collaborating with academic scientists to stimulate "retired" hair follicles and to develop new follicles. One day in the not-too-distant future, we will indeed see products that will eliminate bald spots and restore thick hair.

> Genes have been identified that are important to hair growth. Scientists are studying ways to magnify the "right" signals and block the "wrong" signals to stimulate new hair growth.

STIMULATING EYELASH GROWTH

A new product is available for stimulating eyelash growth. Bimatoprost ophthalmic solution 0.03 percent (Latisse[13]) is now available by prescription for treating hypotrichosis (thinning of eyelashes). This solution has been shown to increase eyelash hair growth, length, thickness, and darkness. It is believed to achieve these results by stimulating the growth phase (anagen phase) of the eyelash hair cycle. The growth phase appears to last longer, with more hairs involved.

Bimatoprost ophthalmic solution, under the brand name Lumigan, has been prescribed for some time by ophthalmologists for glaucoma. Patients putting drops of this solution into their eyes noticed that their eyelashes became thicker and longer, and sometimes their irises became darker. These were listed as risk factors for use of the solution for glaucoma.

Scientists saw the value in developing the solution for eyelash growth. Now Latisse is FDA approved for this use. Contrary to Lumigan, the new product, Latisse, is not applied to the eye itself. Instead, it is applied once nightly to the upper eyelid where the eyelashes emerge from the skin. Since the Latisse solution is not dropped into the eye, the risk of darkening of the iris of the eye is decreased. There is risk, however, that some darkening of the eyelid may occur, which may be reversible if use of the solution is stopped. Potential adverse effects also include itching or redness of the eyes or eyelid. Increased eyelash hair growth will likely not be observed for about two months. Patients with previous eye problems should consult with an ophthalmologist before using the medication.

FAT REMOVAL

Do creams advertised to remove excess fat from thighs and abdomen really work? No cream will reach far enough into skin to do this. There are, however, other alternatives. Exercise and diet are at the top of the list of the best ways to remove excess fat.

There's also liposuction to remove unwanted fat and "sculpture" parts of the body. The dermatologist or plastic surgeon inserts a long hollow tube called a cannula into fat and tunnels it back and forth through the fat cells to destroy, liquefy, and suction up the cells. With liposuction, it is possible to affect one's body shape. But this is not without side effects of blood loss, soreness, and bruising.

New non-invasive alternatives to liposuction are available that make use of high frequency sound waves or lasers to destroy fat cells. "Ultrasonic liposuction"[14] does not require "tunneling" of the cannula.[15] Fat cells are selectively liquefied by the sound waves, leaving surrounding blood vessels, skin, and muscle undamaged. The liquefied fat is broken down and reprocessed by the body or removed by liposuction.

"Body sculpting" lasers[16] specifically target fat cells and destroy them, leaving the skin surface undamaged. Like the ultrasonic devices, these lasers cause fat cells to release fat. The cells and the released fat are then "vacuumed up" by liposuction. These new liposuction techniques are quicker and involve less recovery time than the original liposuction techniques.

> Now available are non-invasive alternatives to liposuction that make use of "body sculpting" lasers or sound waves to destroy fat cells.

DERMAL FILLERS

Tired of those deepening lines around your lips, those deep wrinkles between your nose and mouth? Injections of cow collagen have been around for many years to help plump up wrinkles. Some people, however, are hypersensitive to cow collagen and develop redness and puffiness from the injections.

Human collagen has fewer hypersensitivity reactions. Human collagen was initially obtained from cadavers, however, and having cadaver collagen injected into one's face isn't a pleasant thought.

New "bioengineered" human collagen products are now available that are not derived from cadavers. Instead, they are produced in the lab. CosmoDerm-I NST, CosmoDerm-II NST, and CosmoPlast NST (Inamed Corporation) are injectable human collagen products used similarly to human collagens Zyderm-I, Zyderm-II, and Zyplast, respectively.

Other types of "wrinkle fillers" include Restylane and Juvaderm, hyaluronic acid derivatives. Sculptra, an injectable poly-L-lactic acid product, can "augment tissue",[17] such as cheeks or chins. These fillers can fill

> New "fillers" can fill wrinkles, contour the face, and create better lip definition for a more youthful and attractive appearance.

most deep facial wrinkles, contour the face, and create good lip definition. Effects of Restylane and Juvaderm last four to six months, and effects of Sculptra may last longer.

WARTS

Warts are pesky, persistent growths. Every culture has its own "home remedy" for treating warts. In South Africa, putting the leaf of the banana tree on the wart is reported to work wonders. In the United States, some try duct tape applied to the wart. The dermatologist is likely to treat a wart with liquid nitrogen. This irritates the wart so that it resolves. Often a wart persists without an apparent reaction of the body to get rid of it. When a wart becomes irritated, however, the body takes notice and responds with "skin talk" cytokines to try to eliminate it.

New treatments such as Aldara have emerged that boost the body's own cytokines to treat warts. Another new treatment is 5-aminolevulinic acid (ALA) in combination with PDT. This combination treatment is being tested especially for those hard-to-treat warts on the feet, called "plantar warts." The ALA is applied to a wart, which absorbs the ALA more than the surrounding normal skin. ALA is a potent photosensitizer, which means that it is activated by light to destroy tissue containing the ALA. As the wart is exposed to a certain type of light, the cells making up the wart are destroyed.

ALA in combination with PDT is also being used for treatment of actinic keratoses, those precancerous lesions often found on sun-exposed skin. Studies are also in progress utilizing ALA (injected) and PDT for treatment of skin metastases of breast cancer and other malignancies. ALA and PDT may also be useful for treatment of acne and psoriasis. We will see other exciting uses of this treatment in the near future.

> New wart treatments stimulate the body's own immune system to fight against the wart.

SEBORRHEIC KERATOSES

Like warts, seborrheic keratoses are benign but unattractive growths. These are dark mole-like growths that begin to appear on backs and abdomens of many people in middle and older age. Unlike warts, there's no evidence that seborrheic keratoses are caused by a virus.

ALA in combination with PDT is being tested for treatment of seborrheic keratoses as well as for treatment of warts. In addition, research is ongoing to determine why seborrheic keratoses develop. Studies are in progress to determine the sequence of "skin talk" involved in the development of these growths. This research should lead to treatments to prevent development of these unattractive growths.

> New treatments are in development for elimination and prevention of unsightly age spots called seborrheic keratoses.

ACNE

Oral antibiotics are often used to treat acne patients that have painful acne cysts. But bacteria associated with acne can develop resistance to antibiotics. New treatments for acne are now in development that utilize the body's own resources to reduce inflammation and kill bacteria associated with acne.

Dermcidin is a substance found naturally in sweat gland cells that kills several types of common bacteria and yeast. "Defensins" are small protein fragments produced by skin cells after inflammation. Defensins kill bacteria and yeast. Granulysin, produced by the body's immune cells (T-lymphocytes), kills a variety of bacteria, fungi, and parasites. Scientists are learning how to boost the body's production of these and other substances to kill bacteria and reduce inflammation associated with acne.

> Scientists are harnessing the body's own capabilities to fight acne. They are learning how to enhance the body's own production of substances to kill bacteria and reduce redness, both associated with acne.

The power of light is also being harnessed to treat acne. Lasers are being tested to destroy sebum that clogs pores and results in painful acne cysts. Lasers and IPL can also destroy bacteria that play a role in acne. These bacteria (Propionibacterium acnes) contain "protoporphyrins." Protoporphyrins are substances that can be triggered by laser light to release "singlet oxygen," which causes the bacteria to "self destruct."

New hormone treatments are now approved for treatment of acne. Estrogens,[18] known to be effective in treatment of acne, have rarely been prescribed by dermatologists because of other effects on the body. New FDA-approved, low-dose oral estrogen-containing contraceptives, Estrostep[19] (ethinyl estradiol and norethindrone acetate) and Ortho Tri-Cyclen[20] (norgestimate/ethinyl estradiol), are now available for treatment of acne. These contraceptives decrease the levels of serum free-testosterone, the hormone that contributes to acne breakouts. As with other oral contraceptions, potential risks include blood clots, stroke, and heart attack. These risks are increased by smoking. Contraceptives must not, of course, be taken by women who may be pregnant.

> The power of light is an exciting new treatment for acne. Lasers and IPL devices can kill bacteria associated with acne.

WOUND HEALING

As skin ages, it doesn't heal as quickly from scrapes and cuts as in earlier days. Perhaps the "skin talk" isn't as efficient as before. Perhaps debris that has accumulated within cells over time interferes with "skin talk." Slow wound healing likely results from a combination of factors associated with aging.

Scientists are learning how skin ages and how aging affects wound healing and other skin functions. Cytokines involved in the "skin talk" associated with wound healing are being tested for faster wound healing. New bandages and dressings have been developed to aid in the healing process.

Among these new products are absorptive silver-coated dressings[21] that protect and enhance healing of ulcers and other chronic wounds, new hydrogel dressings that provide an optimum environment for healing skin, Iamin[22] Hydrating Gel, containing a tripeptide-copper ingredient, which allows a wound to retain appropriate moisture while providing a barrier against wound contamination, Regranex [23](beclaplermin) Gel, a topical gel containing a bioengineered platelet-derived growth factor that is useful in treating diabetic foot ulcers.

Bandages containing antibiotics to prevent infection are now available. A word of caution, however. Some individuals may be hypersensitive to some of the antibiotic-containing bandages. For example, some bandages contain Neomycin sulfate, which can cause redness and swelling in individuals sensitive to this product. Stop using any product if it irritates the skin.

Skin substitutes[24] are useful in covering ulcers and other chronic wounds for better healing. Skin substitutes mimic real skin as much as possible, and are often made of cells and other components from real skin. Skin substitutes can be valuable in covering ulcers and other chronic wounds for better healing.

Of course, the best skin substitute would not be just from real skin, but would be from one's *own* skin. EpiDex makes a skin substitute from a person's own hair. Hair from a patient is sent by the patient's physician to the EpiDex company, where cells are cultured[25] to form a graft that can be used as a skin substitute on the patient. Clinical trials are underway for this product.

There are also new ways to close wounds. Calcium alginate has been useful in closing cancer excision sites without sutures. Calcium alginate is derived from seaweed and helps control bleeding, inhibits bacterial growth, and stimulates production of cytokines to heal skin. One downside is that the patient must come back to the office for frequent dressing changes and removal of wound debris.

A medical version of "super glue"[26] is now available in place of a top layer of sutures after skin surgery. It is still necessary for the dermatologist or plastic surgeon to place dissolvable sutures under the skin, but substituting the glue for the top layer of sutures eliminates the suture-induced "railroad tracking" scars. Many physicians still feel more confident applying a top layer of sutures to insure the best "hold" while the skin repairs itself.

> New wound-healing products and wound coverings are available to stimulate more effective wound healing.

NEEDLE-FREE ANESTHETICS

Nobody likes to be stuck by a needle. But if you are having a mole or skin cancer cut out of the skin, you want your skin to be numb! Is there a way to numb the skin without the needle?

Although nothing has yet replaced the effectiveness of injected anesthetic, there are topical anesthetics that are helpful in dulling the pain of injection. EMLA[27] Cream and EMLA Anesthetic Disc (both contain lidocaine 2.5% and prilocaine 2.5%) are (prescription) topical anesthetics for use on normal intact skin for local analgesia. EMLA can be helpful in dulling the pain of Botox injections as well as dulling the pain of injected anesthetics.

EMLA can be used on infants 37 weeks old or more, prior to injection of anesthetic for skin surgery, but it is very important to follow physician recommendations since very serious side effects[28] can occur if left on the skin too long or applied on too large an area.[29] Side effects can include skin blanching, redness, swelling, and itching. EMLA is applied one hour before a procedure. If your child is undergoing a procedure that involves an injection and you are interested in EMLA, discuss with your child's doctor whether EMLA is right for your child.

Fluori-Methane[30] is a topical skin refrigerant used to cool and numb skin prior to injection. Like EMLA, it can diminish discomfort and anxiety from injections. Iontocaine[31], approved by the FDA in May 1996 for dermal surgery on adults and children, utilizes a technique called "iontophoresis" to transfer a water-soluble, charged drug (lidocaine with epinephrine) into the skin. Iontophoresis uses slight electrical currents to transfer medication into skin. Side effects can include skin blanching, redness, and itching, usually transient in nature.

Other needle-free drug delivery systems involve pressurized systems to force liquid medication at high speed through the skin. Others use transdermal gel or liposomes to transport medications across the skin barrier.[32] Industries[33] are working hard to develop mini-needle or needle-free injection systems that will mean less pain with procedures.

> New needle-free injection systems are in development to reduce pain with medical procedures.

TATTOO REMOVAL

Got "Mary loves Joe" tattooed on your arm, and you're in love with Henry? There's hope for you. Tattoos can be removed or made less noticeable by laser surgery or dermabrasion, although scarring may result. Lasers are improving every day, with the ability to target specific substances in skin. The most effective way to remove a tattoo is with lasers that specifically target the individual

> The most effective way to remove a tattoo is with lasers that specifically target the individual colors in a tattoo.

colors in a tattoo. Ask your dermatologist to find a laser center that can do this for you.

HORMONE THERAPY FOR AGING

With aging, there is a decrease in the levels of hormones such as estrogen, testosterone, DHEAS, and growth hormone. Estrogen replacement has been reported to increase skin firmness and elasticity,[34] decrease wrinkling,[35] improve collagen content,[36] enhance vascularization of skin, improve tone and appearance of skin, and enhance hair growth.[37]

These studies suggest that hormone therapy may be beneficial in "turning back the clock." Hormone replacement, however, may have widespread effects in the body, some of which may be beneficial and some of which may be detrimental. Studies continue to determine ways to modify hormones so that they have the desired effect, without having far-reaching, detrimental effects in the body.

> Research is in progress to develop hormones that can be used to enhance skin firmness and decrease wrinkling, while avoiding other effects in the body.

Research is in progress to determine if topical hormone treatments may achieve this goal.

NEEDLE-LESS SCLEROTHERAPY

Lasers and intense pulsed light systems work well for treating tiny blood vessels (telangectasia) on the face. Injecting concentrated saline or other sclerosing agents into veins ("sclerotherapy"), however, is still the "gold standard" for cosmetically treating superficial blood vessels on the legs. But laser companies haven't given up on effectively treating leg veins, and new technologies are in development that should result in effective laser treatment of such veins.

A laser system[38] by Diomed, Inc., has been recently approved by the FDA for treatment of varicose veins, those large, bulging leg veins. The procedure can be done in the doctor's office and involves putting a fiber-optic tip into the vein and slowly withdrawing it while the laser heats and seals the vein shut. We will likely see more treatment of vessels with lasers in the near future.

> New technologies will result in effective laser treatment of leg veins.

COSMETICS TO IMPROVE COMPLEXION

Since time began, women have applied things to their faces to improve their appearance. In ancient times it might have been flour, to lighten the appearance of skin. In Japan, geishas applied a mixture of pigeon dung and other substances to whiten their faces. These substances might have produced the desired appearances but didn't do much for the skin.

Cosmetic companies now recognize that the public has become more discriminating in what is healthy for skin and what is not. Attention is turning towards products that not only improve appearance but also benefit skin.

Cosmetics are often in contact with skin for hours at a time, and can therefore be an excellent conduit for delivering beneficial substances into skin. A cosmetic that can perform such functions is, in reality, a cross between a cosmetic and a pharmaceutical; thus the name, "cosmeceutical."

"Cosmeceuticals" can, for example, incorporate different factors designed to reduce the appearance of fine wrinkles, roughness, sallowness, laxity, hyperpigmentation, and photodamage. Cosmeceuticals can contain antioxidants[39] such as Vitamin C, Vitamin E, and Coenzyme Q10 to minimize free-radical induced skin damage and prevent breakdown of collagen, caused by aging and by

> New "cosmeceuticals" will not only enhance skin appearance but will also treat skin problems.

sunlight. Many of today's cosmeceuticals contain sun protection factors to reduce UVA and UVB exposure. Others can increase dermal collagen synthesis[40] and improve skin thickness, firmness, and elasticity.

Over the years there has been more "hype" than truth in claims that cosmeceuticals "turn back the clock," "erase wrinkles," or "prevent wrinkles." But today's consumer is more savvy and does not believe every claim made. The product must really work to be a success. The pressure is on the manufacturer to produce an effective product. Advertising alone will no longer work.

In the marketplace now are effective skin cleansers that cleanse the skin without damaging the skin barrier.[41] There are moisturizers that repair the skin surface by decreasing water loss.[42] There are sunscreens effective against both UVA and UVB,[43] and there are creams containing antioxidants such as vitamins A, C, and E, as well as plant-derived flavonoids such as soy isoflavones, grape seed extract, and green tea extracts. There are many other creams and lotions containing antioxidants such as Ginkgo extract, rosemary extract, and CoffeeBerry extract.[44] There are pigment lighteners including hydroquinone, Kojic acid (derived from fungus and bacteria), licorice extract, pomegranate extract, and arbutin (derived from the leaves of cranberry and blueberry plants). The list of new cosmeceuticals goes on and on, as demand increases for products to effectively restore and maintain healthy skin.

We are now on the brink of the most exciting time in history for the consumer. As scientists and industries tap into new discoveries by the Genome Project and utilize new technology designed to deliver substances deeper into skin, there will be a wellspring of innovative new cosmeceuticals with truly exciting benefits beyond our wildest dreams.

HOT AREAS OF RESEARCH

- New breakthroughs have led to new mechanisms for treating psoriasis, atopic dermatitis, and skin cancer. Research continues to develop safe and effective treatments.
- Pharmaceutical companies are involved in collaborations to detect and study proteins involved in stimulating the growth phase of the hair cycle.
- Research is in progress to improve the ability of skin to maintain moisture and be protected from environmental stresses.
- Research is in progress to enhance the ability of the dermis to provide a firm foundation for skin.
- Scientists are learning how to increase skin pigment or to decrease skin color.
- The three hottest areas of research in pharmaceutical companies are hair growth, skin pigmentation, and skin aging.

CHAPTER 32

LEARNING FROM THE SIMPLEST ORGANISMS

SECRETS REVEALED BY A TINY WORM

We live in an exciting scientific era with important new discoveries emerging at lightening speed. The past 10 years have seen breakthroughs in scientific discovery beyond the wildest imagination. Yet scientists realize that an infinitesimal number of nature's miracles remain to be discovered.

There are millions of research projects going on this minute, with great potential for new understanding and new therapies. This chapter gives a glimpse into our present-day scientific research, to show where we are and where we are going.

Scientists are a special breed. With relentless curiosity, they peer into microscopes and telescopes, looking at worlds we cannot see. Something catches the scientist's attention, questions arise, and the quest for answers begins. There is a story behind each discovery. One very important story began with a tiny worm, called C. elegans.

The human body is very complex. In the 1950s a group of scientists reasoned that if they could find a simple model to study that had some of the basic characteristics of the human body, they might better understand how the human body works. The scientists became intrigued by the little worm, C. elegans, which has a simple body that includes a brain, nervous system, digestive tract, and reproductive system. Best of all, the worm's "skin" is transparent so that the worm's internal organs can be seen under the microscope.

The scientists found that with the help of the worm, they could understand some puzzling human functions. The scientists published what they discovered, and more scientists began to see the value in studying the simpler systems of the worm to understand the more complicated systems of the human body.

Soon many scientists were sharing new information. Study of the

> Scientists realized that studying the organs of the worm would help them understand how the human body works.

worm's cells and nervous system progressed at full speed. Scientists began finding the worm's genes, and determining the functions of these genes. It soon became possible to predict where, on human DNA, a similar gene with a similar function might be found.

At first, finding genes was a very slow and time-consuming task. Sometimes an entire career was spent looking for a gene. But research was in progress that would result in new technology that would allow rapid detection of genes. With introduction of the new technology, progress in determining the little worm's DNA flew at lightening speed. By mid-1980, the impossible happened—the entire gene sequence of the little worm's DNA was determined!

> By mid-1980, scientists had determined the entire gene sequence of the worm's DNA!

From that point on there was an explosion of productive research. Scientists busily set about determining the functions of the newly discovered genes. They asked, *What happens when a particular gene is missing or turned off? What happens when the gene is overexpressed?* Answers led to knowledge about what a genes does and what it controls.

As scientists continued to study the gene functions in the little worm, other scientists turned to the fruit fly to conduct their research.

SECRETS FROM THE FRUIT FLY

The fruit fly is the little fly that buzzes around the peaches or bananas that have sat in a bowl on the countertop too long. This fly multiplies very rapidly and is therefore an excellent system for studying inherited genes. Scientists found that the DNA of the worm is similar to the DNA of the fly. They also found similarities in the DNA of these creatures to the DNA of humans. As particular genes in the worm and in the fly were studied, therefore, important information about our body's genes emerged.

There were also differences between the DNA of the worm and the fly and that of humans. Scientists studying the fruit fly also noticed that the fly does not have immune cells as we humans have. Immune cells are those cells in our body that rush through the blood stream and out into our tissues to fight bacteria and other invaders. Not only does the fruit fly lack such cells, but it doesn't even have a blood supply to carry such cells, if they were present. Yet the fruit fly seems to be immune from bacterial infection! How can this be? How in the world can a tiny fruit fly escape infection when we humans, with our more sophisticated immune system, are susceptible to bacterial infection?

The question intrigued scientists, who set out on a mission to find the answer. As it turns out, the fruit fly does have an immune system after all—a different system—a very good system. Like little antennae, each cell of the fruit fly has its own "feelers" that project out from its cells. These "feelers," called "Toll-like receptors," are named for the Toll gene that helped them develop. The receptors are able to detect invaders that threaten. Like a toll gate, the Toll-like receptors allow warning signals into the cell.

Once the signal is transmitted inside the fly cell, it is processed so that the cell can respond quickly. Some Toll-like receptors alert the cell to bacteria, others alert to viruses, and others to fungus. When the fly cell receives the signal that a bacteria or fungus is threatening, it responds instantly to attack. Like a ray gun, the cell sprays the invader with toxic substances, knocking holes in the invader's cell membranes. The enemy is vanquished!

What a great system! No need for the cells detecting the invader to run to lymph nodes to alert to the attack. No need for an army of immune cells to return to the scene. No, the cell of the fly is ready right then and there to take up the fight.

It's too bad we don't have a system like that—it's too bad we don't have Toll-like receptors to fight right away on the front lines as the rest of our immune system prepares to fight. As it turns out, we do. The fly helped us find it. By discovering this system in the fly, scientists turned to the human system to look for a similar system, and there it was! Granted, it is better developed in primitive organisms—the sea urchin, for example, has over 100 Toll-like receptors on its cells, whereas only a dozen or so Toll-like receptors have been discovered on human cells. But at least we have such a system, and more receptors on human cells are being discovered each day.

> The fruit fly helped us discover an important aspect of our own immune system.

OUR FIRST LINE OF DEFENSE

What does all of this mean for us? It means that we have a first line of defense that we have inherited, an "innate immune system" that developed along with us as we rose through the evolutionary ranks. It means that our cells begin the battle to protect us, long before our "acquired immune system"—the cells in our blood stream and in our tissues that protect us—kicks in. It means that our little cells have their own defense. When they sense a threat, they produce antithreat substances, they punch holes in the threatening organism, and they spew out signals to alert our "acquired immune system."

But our primitive system doesn't stand alone. In addition to providing a "front-line attack," it also interfaces with our more sophisticated immune system, the acquired immune system. The signals spewed out are received by "dendritic cells," little messenger cells that rush to the lymph nodes where they alert immune cells to come to the attack.

The growing knowledge of our innate immune system, our first line of defense, raises the question of whether we can help boost our cells' production of the substances that punch holes in the threatening organisms and alert our acquired immune system. Scientists are study-

> A new frontier in fighting infection and cancer is helping to boost our body's own defense mechanisms that respond to these threats.

ing ways to stimulate more production of such substances, either by stimulating our cells or by bioengineering these substances. In these ways, we may be able to boost our defenses one hundred fold.

POSSIBLE NEW TREATMENTS FOR AUTOIMMUNE DISORDERS

What if the immune response is overactive? An overactive response occurs in "autoimmune" disorders such as lupus or multiple sclerosis. In such disorders, a mistake happens. Normal cells mistakenly signal danger to the Toll-like receptors. This results in the cell thinking there is an invader, when there isn't. Immune cells rush to the rescue, creating inflammation and damage to normal tissues, when this shouldn't have happened.

Study of Toll-like receptors of the fruit fly has generated ideas for treatment of such "autoimmune" disorders. By blocking such mistaken signals to the receptors, we may be better able to prevent the damage. This type of "signal blocking" may also be useful in preventing heart, lung, or kidney transplant rejection.

ANTICANCER POSSIBILITIES

If our cells can detect invading bacteria and other organisms, can they also detect cells that have become cancerous? The answer is yes. Our cells can indeed detect cancer. Certain Toll-like receptors or normal cells detect cancerous cells and transmit this information inside the normal cell.

If our cells can detect cancer cells and transmit this warning to our immune cells, why don't our immune cells rush to attack the cancer cells? As it turns out, a cancer cell can trick the attack cells into thinking that it is a normal cell. Although the Toll-like receptor is telling the attack cells to kill, the cancer cell is signaling to the attack cells, "I'm normal; don't damage me." This masquerade allows the cancer cell to continue to grow and to do its damage.

Is there a way to remedy this deceit? Can the attack cells be shown that the cancer cells are only disguising themselves as normal cells but are, in truth, the enemy? This idea has led to ongoing "cancer vaccine" tests at the National Institute of Health to try to make the dendrite cells more excited, to stimulate more attack cells that recognize the cancer cells for what they are, and to boost production of substances toxic to the cancer cells.

Now that scientists are learning more about how these signals work and the sinister nature of cancer cells, they are designing ways to "tweak" the Toll-like receptors and the attack system to get better results.

The FDA has already approved imiquimod cream (Aldara), which stimulates a Toll-like receptor (TLR7), for treatment of superficial basal cell skin cancer.[1]

Other therapies are not far behind as scientists observe the world around us, ask questions, and seek answers.

> Breaking the genetic code of the tiny worm has led to the breaking of the human DNA code.

LOOKING TO THE FUTURE

These are only a few glimpses into current research of nature's tiny creatures that is leading to exciting new medical therapies. What we have learned from the tiny worm and the fruit fly is leading to new and exciting therapies for infection, cancer, and other problems. Most exciting of all is that breaking the genetic code of the tiny worm has now led, in this century, to the breaking of the human DNA code. We have entered an exciting "new genomic era" that is bringing innovative new products and therapies to skin care.

CHAPTER 33

THE NEW GENOMIC ERA— HOW IT WILL IMPACT SKIN CARE

Not so long ago, a scientist might have spent a lifetime discovering and studying the unique code that makes up one particular gene. Genes are found within the DNA (deoxyribonucleic acid) of all cells, so when we refer to "one gene," we are referring to a gene that is present in every cell of the body. But there are over 20,000 genes in our DNA. To discover and understand the code and sequence of all of these genes seemed an impossible task, even for several lifetimes.

In 2003, the astounding announcement was made to the world that the human gene had been sequenced. This meant that for the first time scientists had determined the alphabet code for every gene that makes up the human body!

Scientists are now discovering what these different genes do and how they perform. They are discovering abnormalities in genes that cause medical problems[1]. They are discovering how genes function to keep the body operating normally.

Each gene is made up of a long sequence of nucleotides. One tiny change in a normal gene may cause tumors to grow, blood cells to multiply out of control, uncontrolled bleeding or clotting to occur, or many other abnormal situations to develop. A gene change may be inherited, or it may occur as a spontaneous mutation caused by a virus or other factor. Sometimes a change in only one gene may cause the problem. At other times several genes may be involved.

> Scientists have now done what a generation before us thought impossible—they have determined the alphabet code for every gene that makes up the human body!

If a gene abnormality is inherited, every cell may be affected. For example, "albinism," or loss of color in skin, can be caused by an inherited gene disorder. Persons with certain types of albinism are born without the necessary gene to produce skin pigment. Their skin is white and susceptible to severe sunburn and development of skin cancers. If we could replace the faulty gene with a normal gene, skin could be restored to its normal color.

If a gene abnormality is acquired after birth, only a cluster of cells may be affected. Excessive sun exposure, for example, results in gene changes that can lead to skin cancer. Radiation from the sun penetrates cells and damages genes. The body attempts to repair the damage, and when all works well, the damaged part of the gene is spiced out and a repaired part inserted. When this

> If defective genes that cause defects and diseases could be replaced by normal genes, we would be able to treat many untreatable conditions. But there are still many problems to be solved before gene therapy becomes a practical treatment.

repair system breaks down or is overwhelmed, cells with damaged genes may multiply uncontrollably to result in skin cancer. As scientists learn the "skin talk" necessary for gene repair, we may have new gene therapies in the future that will assist in such repair.

GENE THERAPY

There are many problems that could be treated, in theory, with "gene therapy." But there are huge challenges before gene therapy becomes useful and safe.

First, scientists must understand what gene is defective. Then they must understand what other genes interact with the defective gene. Does replacing the gene solve the problem? Or does it create other problems?

Second, scientists must find a way to correct the gene in all relevant cells. Repairing the gene in one or a cluster of cells won't do the job if many cells have the defective gene.

Third, how can the gene be repaired? A virus is often used. The repaired parts are attached to the DNA or RNA[2] of a virus, which can get into cells. The virus, with the attached repair mechanism, penetrates the cell. Once inside, the repair mechanism is released to do its job. This process can be tricky. Only a few cells may be affected. Or the virus may not release the repair mechanism, causing damage. Finally, the best viruses for getting a gene into a cell are potentially cancer-causing. Other, safer viruses are being checked for transferring genes into cells.

There's a long road yet to travel in developing gene therapy that is safe and effective, but scientists are hard at work on this problem and are making strides every day.

NEW APPROACHES

Expression of genes results in "gene products," such as proteins or other molecules. The study of what specific genes actually produce and what these molecules do is called "functional genomics." "Proteomics" is the study of proteins expressed by genes. These are currently very "hot" areas of research.

> Gene therapy in the future will give us exciting new therapies to combat disease and aging.

A defective gene is likely to produce defective "gene products." Defective gene products may result in many abnormal functions, such as cells multiplying when they shouldn't, or cells dying when they shouldn't.

Another approach to gene therapy is to correct the gene products rather than the gene itself. As scientists learn what proteins and other molecules are produced by different genes, these proteins and molecules can be blocked or enhanced, depending upon what is needed for normal functioning of the gene. It also may be possible to supply molecules that should be produced by the abnormal gene. These new areas of research will result in exciting new therapies to combat disease and aging.

Preliminary research shows that delivering certain enzyme proteins into skin can help treat certain genetic disorders affecting skin. For example, Xeroderma pigmentosa is an inherited skin condition that results in numerous skin cancers because of the lack of an important enzyme that repairs DNA damaged by exposure to the sun. Scientists are working to develop a system for replacing the missing enzyme to treat this condition.

AN INCREDIBLE ERA IN SKIN CARE

We are now entering the most incredible era in skin care and medical therapy. Not only are scientists detecting genes that determine our characteristics, our disease susceptibilities, our drug reactions, and many other personal features. They are also finding out how our genes function.

As we learn more and more about skin, its components and interactions, we are finding ways to improve health and treat diseases, and we are finding ways to combat skin aging, grow hair, and look healthier and more attractive.

Gene research is vast in scope and progressing at a rapid pace. Scientists are learning what causes genes to be activated and repressed. They are identifying proteins expressed by genes that are important in carrying out the gene instructions. They are learning how certain cells respond to these proteins. They are discovering an intricate and complex set of interactions of genes and proteins. By studying genes, scientists are learning how different functions of the body can be delicately manipulated for specific treatments.

Important strides have been made. Genetic testing is available for determining whether individuals carry genes associated with certain inherited disorders. Information learned from such testing may predict whether an individual is at increased risk of developing a certain inherited disorder and whether he or she is likely to pass the trait to offspring. The DNA in any one human is 99.9 percent like that of other humans. However, the .1 percent difference can determine whether someone may develop heart problems, mental problems, diabetes, or other medical problems.

Gene studies are also leading to the potential for predicting susceptibility to certain diseases and to developing "designer drugs." Imagine learning exactly how you will react to a certain medication, or whether a medication will be effective for the particular type of a disease that you have. Imagine having your medication for treatment of a potential disorder specifically tailored to you. This is work in progress.

Small "snippets"[3] of DNA are also being investigated for associations with susceptibility to certain diseases, with reactions to certain medications, and with effectiveness of medications for particular conditions. The HapMap Gene Project is an ongoing project involving more than 200 scientists from around the world, all of whom are working together to determine differences in DNA that correspond with different medical problems or drug sensitivities. They aim to make a "road map" for detecting susceptibilities in individuals.[4]

Your skin will benefit from these exciting projects, as will your overall health. The future holds effective technological analysis of your skin so that skin treatments can be designed specifically for you. The future also holds promise of treatment of genetic disorders that have been untreatable in the past.

Keep abreast with what is new through government and academic Web sites. Talk to your dermatologist. The truth is that breakthroughs arise not from advertising hype but from scientific discovery—and from putting the pieces together to reveal opportunities for translation of those discoveries into breakthrough products.

CHAPTER 34

RENEWING OUR BODY: STEM CELLS AND TISSUE TRANSPLANTATION

OUR SELF-RENEWING STEM CELLS

Most cells in the body have reached their destiny. These are skin cells, blood cells, liver cells, muscle cells, nerve cells, brain cells, heart cells, and many others. They perform their jobs and when they become "worn out," they die and are replaced by similar specialized, or "differentiated" cells.

> Stem cells are our "self-renewing" cells that generate new cells to replace the old.

The cells that gave birth to these cells are called "stem cells." These are our "self-renewing" cells. They are found within skin, within bone marrow where blood cells are born, within the liver—within all specialized tissues. They are there to generate new cells to replace the old.

Stem cells still maintain full potential to differentiate into specialized cells. They are termed, "adult stem cells" or "somatic stem cells." They are rather hard to identify in tissue, but scientists are learning more ways to identify them. Scientists are now able to take adult stem cells, put them in a culture dish, and induce them to multiply.

The multiplied product can be very useful in replacing damaged tissues. For example, sheets of skin cells grown from stem cells can be placed over wounds for better healing. Adult stem cells also have the potential to grow new hair, repair various tissues inside the body, and treat diabetes and many other diseases.

Adult stem cells tend to produce cells like those around them. Stem cells in the skin tend to give birth to skin cells. Stem cells in the bone marrow, where blood cells are produced, tend to give birth to blood cells. Stem cells in muscle tend to produce muscle cells. Recent research, however, has shown that under certain conditions, adult stem cells can form other types of cells.

"Embryonic stem cells" (cells from an embryo) are more versatile and can differentiate into *any* of the cells in the human body. Embryonic stem cells multiply easily. These stem cells are potentially valuable not only in repairing tissue but also in developing new organs. There is great hope for using embryonic stem cells to treat debilitating disorders such as Alzheimers, Parkinson's, heart disease, spinal cord injury, and vision and hearing loss.

> Stem cells have great potential in replacing damaged cells. Research on stem cells can lead to treatments for conditions such as spinal cord injury, heart disease, Parkinson's, and Alzheimers.

Most early research on stem cells was done in the mouse. Scientists worked with stem cells from embryos and from adults, first in the mouse and then with human stem cells. Most human embryos used for research were obtained from "in vitro fertilization" clinics where excess embryos were not used and were about to be discarded. They were donated for research with the consent of the donor.

Vigorous controversy arose, however, over the use of human embryos in research. Not only were people concerned about destruction of the embryos, but they were also concerned about implications of human cloning. In 2001, the Bush administration[1] imposed a ban on embryonic stem cell research.

Unable to continue their research on human embryos, scientists turned their attention to adult stem cells. Perhaps, they reasoned, adult stem cells could be isolated from skin and reprogrammed "back in time" into precursor stem cells that would act like embryonic stem cells.

They were successful. Researchers in two labs, one in Japan[2] and another in Wisconsin,[3] showed that normal human skin cells can be reprogrammed into cells called "induced pluripotent stem cells" (iPS), that act like embryonic stem cells. This miraculous achievement was accomplished by inserting four genes[4] into the skin cells. These genes, important in early development in the embryo, converted the cells back into cells that acted like embryonic stem cells.

> Scientists have found that stem cells from one organ of the body can be "reprogrammed" into cells from another organ of the body.

Scientists showed that stem cells from skin,[5] "reprogrammed" in this way, have the remarkable capacity to form not only new skin, but also other types of tissues. This suggested the exciting possibility that scientists might be able to "reprogram" stem cells from skin to grow new tissue for other parts of the body.

Developing the iPS was a great step forward. The potential was now present for taking a sample of a patient's skin, converting the cells to iPS, then inducing the cells to become whatever tissue was needed for repair in the patient. Scientists tested this potential in highly successful experiments.

Lou Gehrig's disease, or ALS (amyotrophic lateral sclerosis) is a progressive condition where motor nerve cells die. Motor nerve cells transmit messages from the spinal cord to the body's muscles. Death of these nerve cells leads to paralysis. In 2008, researchers from Harvard and Columbia University took skin cells from an 82-year-old woman with Lou Gehrig's disease. The researchers were able to entice these skin cells to transform into motor nerve cells![6]

In diabetes, insulin-producing "beta cells"[7] die in the pancreas. In 2008, a research team from the Harvard Stem Cell Institute took enzyme-producing cells in the pancreas of a mouse and turned them into beta cells that produced insulin! Cells that once produced gut enzymes to digest food were now producing insulin to regulate blood sugar.

In February 2009, scientists from the University of Wisconsin-Madison were able to convert human skin cells into beating heart muscle cells. These experiments furnished further proof that cells from one part of the body can be transformed into cells from another part of the body.

Much more research is needed before these research accomplishments can be turned into treatments. Many experiments are performed in the mouse or in culture dishes, with clinical trials in humans yet to come. But results continue to be encouraging, and research is progressing at a rapid pace. Cells have now been reprogrammed from many other organs such as liver, stomach, and brain into many different kinds of cells in the body.

There are still important hurdles to overcome. To transform cells into iPS involves four genes, one[8] of which is cancer-causing. In addition, the virus[9] used to transport these genes into the cells is cancer-causing. The iPS cells are still modified cells and just how close they are to true embryonic cells is not certain. The genes used to transform cells into iPS can land anywhere in the cell during transfer, adding to the risk of cancerous changes.

Scientists are meeting the challenges. It is now possible to make iPS using only the three non-carcinogenic genes. A less carcinogenic virus[10] has been found to insert genes into the cells. Yet concerns of carcinogenesis remain; more must be learned about "skin signals" that direct a cell and its tissue to develop in a healthy manner. Research on embryonic stem cells would bypass many of the hurdles presented by using iPS cells.

In March 2009, President Obama lifted the ban on embryonic stem cell research, allowing this important research to proceed. The Department of Health and Human Services is developing ethical and reporting guidelines for stem cell research to address concerns of the ethical issues surrounding use of embryonic stem cells in research. The future holds promise of new therapies of enormous potential for saving lives, generating new organs, and treating previously untreatable disorders.

Stem cell research offers possibilities for treating spinal cord injuries, replacing damaged cells that perform important functions, and treating previously untreatable disorders.

CHAPTER 35

TISSUE ENGINEERING — MAKING A NEW BODY PART

Organ transplants save millions of lives every day. But the system needs improvement. The waiting list is long for transplanted organs, and many people die before they can get their transplant. Transplantation normally requires immunosuppressive medications that can create other complications. Rejections can occur.

Scientists are working hard to come up with another alternative—one that sounds like science fiction, but is real. They are "constructing" organs with living cells.[1] They are making new body parts.

Is this possible? In 1995, Joseph Vacanti, M.D., pioneer in tissue engineering, showed that it is possible. He constructed a human ear on the back of a mouse. How did he do this? He molded a scaffold in the shape of an ear, using a biodegradable substance (a substance that the body will eventually dissolve). Over this scaffold, he "planted" skin cells. The scaffold was attached to the back of a mouse so that there would be a blood supply. The cells multiplied to cover the scaffold, which was still in the shape of an ear. Eventually the scaffold dissolved (was "biodegraded"), and an ear remained.

It wasn't a perfect ear, however. It didn't have its own blood supply to nourish it—it had to borrow from the mouse. So work is in progress to create a blood supply for the ear and to develop other organs constructed in a similar manner.

Scientists are working on engineering livers, kidneys, and other organs by "planting" skin cells over the biodegradable scaffolds. The key is in using the right cells—those that do have the capacity to turn into any kind of cell of the body—and the right signals ("skin talk"). The right cells, as we have learned from the previous chapter, are stem cells.

Embryonic stem cells can be transformed into any desired tissue type by developing a suitable "scaffolding" for the cells to grow and by having the right "mix" of cell signals in the environment surrounding the cells. The scaffolding provides a structure that physically coaxes the cells into the right configuration. The cell signals induce the stem cells to form the correct tissue or organ. Scientists are designing new, intricate nanoscale scaffolds and determining appropriate signals to send to certain cells so that cells will differentiate appropriately and blood vessels will form where needed.

> Scientists are well on their way towards constructing new organs for transplantation.

This research is leading to the development of renewed tissue and organs for transplantation. Imagine a biocompatible "liver" constructed to help the patient until a liver transplant is possible. Or a new heart valve to replace a damaged one. Imagine skin coaxed into making a new nose for those with severe nose injuries—or a new hand, or other part of the body. Science fiction? No—it's work in hot progress now.

Already available is Epicel, a permanent skin replacement grown from the patient's own skin cells. This "epidermal sheet" of cells can help heal burns. Also available is Carticel, an injectable suspension of chrondrocytes (cartilage cells) for repairing cartilage. Vascugel is a blood vessel patch which, like a large cellular bandage, is placed on top of a damaged blood vessel to send signals to promote healing of the vessel. At least 70 companies are now developing tissue-engineered products for implantation, including skin used for grafts, large bioengineered blood vessels, and other implants to replace a patient's damaged tissue.[2]

Whole organs are not far behind. In development are an engineered liver, bone, bladder, and heart muscle. Scientists[3] pushing the forefront of tissue engineering are utilizing new nanotechnology, developments in stem cell biology, and discoveries in cell signaling to make incredible strides in bringing tissue engineering from the laboratory to the bedside to save lives.

CHAPTER 36

NANOTECHNOLOGY — A WHOLE NEW WORLD

W e live in our own plane of existence. But the Hubble telescope has confirmed for us that there is a much larger dimension of planets, stars, and galaxies in this magnificent Universe. Likewise, there are smaller dimensions. We can see the diameter of a hair—that is about 1,000 nanometers (nm) wide. But we can't see much smaller than that. We can't see cells or bacteria with the naked eye, and we certainly can't see the tiny universe of protons, atoms, electrons, neutrons, and molecules. Now there are new entities to contemplate. Chemists and other scientists have created a wide variety of incredibly tiny nanoparticles, just a little larger than an atom. Why would they want to create something so small—that they couldn't see? Scientists have learned that these tiny particles have enormous potential for health and beauty.

Imagine tiny capsules so small that they *could* squeeze through the skin and travel down deep enough to take substances to fibroblasts to stimulate production of new collagen or elastin, eliminating wrinkles and making skin firm. Imagine tiny vessels seeking out stem cells to deliver certain stimulatory substances, making baby-like skin. Imagine these vessels delivering substances to stimulate inactive hair follicles to grow hair again. Imagine tiny nanorobots[1] swimming through the bloodstream to fight disease at its source. But these are not just for the imagination. These are real projects in development today.

Nanoparticles are incredibly small particles—only a little larger than an atom. They are so small, they can penetrate into the skin.

Nanoparticles range from 1 nm to 100 nm. They are just a little larger than an atom, which ranges from 0.1 to 0.5 nanometers (nm) in diameter. They are so small they can indeed penetrate through the skin.

We know from earlier chapters that most creams and lotions that are advertised to clear wrinkles may moisturize, and thereby help fine wrinkles, but they do not penetrate deep enough into skin to affect deep wrinkles. But the tiny nanoparticles have the potential to pass right through the skin barriers that prevent creams and lotions from entering the skin. And they can be constructed to deliver substances into the skin.

Scientists have learned that nanoparticles behave differently than larger particles. As a particle becomes smaller, the ratio of its surface to its volume grows. This makes the surface more available, and therefore more powerful, for interacting with skin components or with other nanoparticles.

A new tiny arsenal of nanoparticles for every imaginable purpose has been developed in recent years by chemists, physicists, physicians, and engineers. Chemists from Rice University[2] developed a "car" no larger than a molecule with four carbon molecules shaped like soccer balls. The car moves by the random collisions of the molecules around them ("Brownian motion"). In 2004, a research team from Pennsylvania State University[3] developed little nanometers that moved by converting energy stored in certain fuel molecules. In 2002, a research team from Harvard University[4] developed a nanoscale "boat" that spontaneously moves on the surface of a tank of water containing hydrogen peroxide. Bubbles of oxygen from the disintegration of the hydrogen peroxide pushed the boat forward, like jet propulsion. More recently, scientists have shown that nanoparticles can be driven by light. Reactions of the light on molecules result in energy that moves the nanoparticle. Other scientists are working on electric fields to move molecules.

Why all this research on moving a nanoparticle? It is not an idle hobby. There are thousands of practical applications. In the field of medicine, such tiny machines could move towards a target, a tumor or infection, for example, delivering a payload to destroy the problem.

Besides creating nanoparticles that move, scientists are working on how to "target" the nanoparticle to a desired location, such as a tumor or infection. How do you tell the nanoparticle that this tumor, for example, is your target—not that normal cell next to it? This is where the scientists come into play that are studying Toll-like receptors and cell signals ("skin talk") and immune cells of the body. These scientists are learning what cellular structures or what cell signals distinguish cancerous cells or infections from normal cells and normal tissue. These scientists are designing ways to "entice" the moving nanomachines to the correct locations to deliver their payloads.

> Nanoparticles bring the possibility of developing exciting new ways to deliver active ingredients deep down into skin—past the skin barrier, even through the basement membrane and into the dermis where collagen and elastin provide skin support. There is now hope for delivering cytokines and other "skin talk" signals down into the dermis to stimulate more collagen and elastin, making skin firmer, with fewer wrinkles. Likewise, antioxidants could be incorporated into nanoparticles and delivered deep into skin to prevent disruption of collagen and elastin, preserving firm skin.

What sort of payload could "nanomachines" deliver? The nanoparticles may be constructed to be solid or hollow to contain a substance to be delivered into skin. At the University of Texas, scientists are using mice to explore the use of gold nanoparticles to increase destruction of melanoma by infrared light. Infrared light generates heat that can destroy mouse melanoma cells, but good tissue is destroyed as well by the heat. The nanoparticles are targeted to, and penetrate, the melanoma cells. A low dose of infrared light is used, too low to kill normal tissue but enough to heat up the gold nanoparticles inside the melanoma, killing the cells.

Scientists at the Penn State College of Medicine use another payload to treat melanoma. They are using small bits of RNA (siRNA) within lipid-based nanoparticles to attack cancer-causing genes within melanoma cells in mice. They use an ultrasound device to create microscopic holes in the skin surface, allowing the nanoparticles to leak into the tumor cells beneath the skin, inactivating the cancer-causing genes and shrinking the tumors.

Scientists at the Georgia Institute of Technology are targeting "magnetic nanoparticles" to human ovarian cancer cells implanted in the mouse. The scientists pass a magnet over the skin surface and "lift" the cancer cells close to the skin surface so that they can be removed.

Other scientists are using nanoparticles to detect diseased tissue. Scientists at the Georgia Institute of Technology and Emory University have developed a nanoparticle that can detect trace amounts of hydrogen peroxide in animals. Hydrogen peroxide is believed to be overproduced by cells in certain early disease states. When the nanoparticle detects hydrogen peroxide within the animal, the nanoparticle emits light that can be detected by certain instruments, alerting the doctor to the possibility of early disease.

These are only a few examples of the many research projects involving the use of nanoparticles to target and destroy cancers and detect diseases. These experiments are in mice and are far from being ready for use in humans, but they illustrate the new frontier of translating what is discovered in the laboratory into useful medical therapies.

What about nanoparticles for skin care and skin problems? You will hear more and more about nanoparticles, picoparticles (even smaller than nanoparticles), nanoemulsions (tiny oil and water emulsions for delivery of substances into skin), fullerenes (tiny molecular "cages" for transporting substances into skin), and nanodevices (such as tiny "robots" to perform a task like attacking a skin tumor). Although nanotechnology is still in early stages, many new moisturizers, sunscreens, cleansers, and acne medications incorporating this technology are already in the marketplace. These products in general are usually easy to apply and disperse easily onto skin, giving good protection of the skin surface.

There are still safety issues to determine—for example, if a desired substance is delivered deep into skin, will the desired effect be the only effect—or will there be a cascade of other unwanted effects? Since there are still debates and concerns about these issues, some companies already using nanoparticles have not yet advertised their products as such.

> Nanotechnology is bringing a whole new meaning to "cosmeceuticals." Now there is great potential for utilizing scientific discovery in new skin care products and treatments.

The prospect for putting into practical use the new discoveries involving skin signals, gene functions, and stem cells is tremendously exciting. But there is always risk of advertising hype rather than truth. "Nanoparticle" can easily become just another buzz word. A claim that some rare plant or beetle juice is encapsulated in a nanoparticle to make skin younger still suggests advertising hype. It's the science behind a product that counts. Look for the proof. Do your research. Ask your doctor. The technology is available to make exciting changes. Time will tell if product claims are true or are mere promises.

So while today's cosmetic advertisements may promise more than is delivered, a whole new world of nanocosmetics and nanotherapies is emerging where our wildest dreams *can* come true. As we continue to separate hype from truth, the future holds astounding opportunities for renewed beauty, youth, and health!

CHAPTER 37

MEDICAL TOURISM — A VACATION AND A FACE LIFT?

A re the wrinkles in your face getting you down? Is your face sagging like a hound dog? Do you want to look years younger but not let anyone know that you are planning a face lift? Do you want to go on vacation and come back *really* looking refreshed?

"Medical tourism" is a concept resounding around the world. Countries looking for new sources of income and trade are capitalizing on the big demand for good, but affordable, health and cosmetic care.

Let's face it. We all want to look good. There is a huge body of consumers that wants to turn back the clock and improve appearance. There are the baby boomers. There are those in the work place who feel that looking their best will enhance their job competitiveness. There are those who simply want to look good.

Spas expanded in number to accommodate the increased demand for cosmetic services. As lasers and other complex technologies became available, medical offices expanded their services to accommodate demand for cosmetic practices. Some academic institutions promoted the concept of "appearance centers," where a person wanting to look and feel better could come to a center for evaluation and referral to the appropriate specialists within the institution for addressing all appearance and health problems.

Foreign and domestic industry also realized the potential of advertising medical centers. Now over 50 countries consider medical tourism one of their industries. Many people would love to have a procedure done privately away from home and perhaps take a trip at the same time.

> You can take a vacation to an exotic place and have a face lift at the same time.

Medical tourism has become increasingly popular in recent years as people look for high-quality procedures that they can afford. There are good financial deals in some foreign countries. Many medical and cosmetic treatments are available, depending upon the facility. These may include plastic surgery, cosmetic procedures, liver transplantation, orthopedic surgery, heart surgery, and others.

Some insurance policies may cover treatment abroad if the problem is not considered cosmetic. The wait time for procedures is likely to be short, and the level of personal care high. Many of the physicians involved have trained in well-known places, and excellent care can be found. *But* not all facilities are alike—accreditation and quality assurance can vary widely, creating risks.

If you are considering going abroad for cosmetic or other treatment, it is important to consult your own physician for recommendations. Some of the United States' best hospitals have affiliations or satellite facilities abroad and can give advice.

CHAPTER 38

TAKING TECHNOLOGY HOME

Tired of shaving legs and underarms? Don't want the trouble of depilatories or the pain of waxing? Can't afford the time or money to go to a spa or medical office for a laser hair removal? You are in luck. The FDA has approved an at-home laser hair removal device. You will see more and more at-home devices previously found only in spas or medical facilities.

At-home laser hair removal devices, such as the Tria, can be somewhat expensive (around $1,000), but you would spend that much anyway on a sequence of in-office laser treatments sufficient to remove hair.

Hair grows in cycles. Lasers target dark hair follicles. Dark hair follicles are more predominant in the growing (anagen) phase of the hair cycle rather than the resting or falling out phases of the cycle. Therefore the hairs in the growing phase are going to respond best to laser treatment, and those in the resting and the falling out phases are likely going to need repeat treatment. Rather than spend those extra visits in-office, you can now laser at home. At first, treatments will need to be every few weeks, then less frequently.

There are downsides. There may be skin irritation. Dark-skinned individuals can lose skin color and should not use current at-home laser treatments. The laser won't work on red, blonde, or gray hair since there is no dark hair follicle. If you are considering an at-home laser, discuss this first with your physician.

> Laser hair removal can now be done at home.

At-home low-lever laser "combs" and other treatments for hair loss and psoriasis are also emerging into the marketplace. Look for new technologies not only in the medical offices and spas but also for use at home. Look for FDA approval and check with your physician before purchasing.

CHAPTER 39

THE CASE FOR VITAMIN D

Vitamin D_3 (cholecalciferol) is generated in skin when light is absorbed by a molecule in skin, 7-dehydrocholesterol. People need some sunlight for this reaction to occur. There are also dietary sources of Vitamin D, including fish oil, egg yolk, and various plants. Plants contain Vitamin D_2 (ergosterol).

A normal diet does not usually contain enough Vitamin D. Sufficient exposure to sunlight or Vitamin D supplements are therefore necessary. Vitamin D is converted by the liver into 25-hydroxycholecalciferol and into 1,25-dihydroxycholecalciferol, the active form, in the kidney.

Vitamin D helps the intestine absorb calcium and provides a correct balance of calcium and phosphorous, important for strong bones and teeth. But this is not all that it does. Almost all cells in the body have receptors for Vitamin D. This means that Vitamin D affects virtually all of our body. In skin, it appears important in cell differentiation and proliferation. Cell differentiation is important in the development of the skin layers as new skin cells migrate upwards to the skin surface. Proliferation, or multiplication of cells, is important in the "birthing" of new skin cells for skin renewal and to replace worn-out cells.

The National Center for Health Statistics estimates that at least 36 percent of all Americans are deficient in Vitamin D. Effects of Vitamin D deficiency emphasize the importance of gaining enough of this vitamin. The effect on bone mineralization can be seen in pictures of rickets, where the legs and arms of children with this deficiency are bowed. Vitamin D deficiency can also contribute to other health problems such as osteoporosis, depression, autoimmune diseases, and cancer.

Sunscreens can block Vitamin D synthesis in skin, yet without sunscreen there is risk of skin cancer and photoaging. What is the answer?

Wearing sunscreen will decrease the skin's production of Vitamin D. Vitamin D deficiency is a great risk for those who are housebound, without any sun exposure, and with poor diets. But the AAD estimates that more than a million new cases of skin cancer will be diagnosed in the United States this year and that many studies have found an association between sunburns and increased risk of melanoma. The AAD recommends that everyone wear a sunscreen with at least SPF 15 year-round and get vitamin D safely through a healthy diet that may include vitamin supplements. In the United States and in most developed countries, many foods contain supplemental Vitamin D.

> Wear sunscreen to protect from the sun and get vitamin D safely through a healthy diet that may include vitamin supplements.

The AAD also recommends that those who are concerned about not getting enough Vitamin D should discuss this with their doctors. Your Vitamin D levels can be checked and appropriate supplementation as necessary can be prescribed.

Is there such a thing as too much Vitamin D? Yes. Too much can be toxic. If a supplement is suggested, follow your doctor's recommendations.

CHAPTER 40

THE FINISHING TOUCH

In 2009 an overweight, frumpy woman stepped onto the stage of the show, *Britain's Got Talent*. Her eyebrows were thick and bushy, her dress was dowdy, her hair was loose and unstyled. The panel of judges sat back with smirks on their faces. Surely this was a joke. They prepared themselves for some corny singing—ready for the occasional leg-pulling that is seen on such shows.

Within seconds, the judges' eyebrows lifted and smiles of wonder appeared on their faces as the most beautiful voice emerged. The frumpy woman now appeared miraculously beautiful during her performance. Her confidence shown through as she sang, her eyes sparkled, her smile was genuine. The performance of Susan Doyle was one of the most watched You Tube events of all times.

To see someone transformed during such a moment is a poignant reminder that beauty lies within. Her beauty emerged when her wondrous voice came forth. She knew her talent and the audience felt her joy in sharing her song. When you think of how you want to find the fountain of youth for your skin, when you think how you may banish wrinkles with Botox, fill in facial creases with fillers, polish the surface of your skin with chemical peels and microdermabrasion, even skin color with laser and intense pulsed light, use new nano-creams to firm skin and create a youthful appearance, think of Susan Doyle. Compare her to the plastic faces of those who have tried too hard to perfect their appearances. Remember that true beauty lies within, and that unless your face projects that inner beauty, you will not achieve what you seek.

Going too far can create a plastic look—expressions frozen by too much Botox, lips exaggerated out of proportion, faces sanded and lasered until no color remains. Look alive, smile, reflect inner happiness, and confidence. And you are beautiful!

APPENDIX

DERMATOLOGY ORGANIZATIONS

- The American Academy of Dermatology: www.aad.org.

DERMATOLOGY PUBLICATIONS

- *The Journal of the American Academy of Dermatology*: (www.eblue.org)
- *Archives of Dermatology*: http://archderm.ama-assn.org/
- *The International Journal of Dermatology*: see www.blackwell-science. com/
- *Cutis*: www.cutis.com
- *Cosmetic Dermatology*: www.cosderm.com/index.htm
- *Dermatology Times*: www.dermatologytimes.com/dermatologytimes/

SKIN CARE, DERMATOLOGICAL PROBLEMS AND PROCEDURES

- SkinCarePhysicians.com (www.skincarephysicians.com) provides patients with information on treatment and management of skin diseases, including psoriasis, eczema, aging skin, acne, melanoma, and actinic keratoses.
- For more information about and pictures of benign lesions, precancerous lesions, skin cancers, Mohs micrographic surgery, and other dermatological surgery procedures, see the Loyola University Dermatology Medical Education Web site at http://www.meddean.luc.edu/lumen/ MedEd/medicine/dermatology/melton/title.htm.
- For answers to common dermatological questions, see http:// www.medhelp.org/forums/dermatology/wwwboard.html.
- An excellent site for information about skin problems as well as other medical problems is Harvard Medical School's Consumer Health Information site at http://www.intelihealth.com/IH/ihtIH/WSIHW000/ 408/408.html.

- For information about cosmetic procedures, see The American Academy of Facial Plastic and Reconstructive Surgery at www .aafprs.org/. See also:http://www.plasticsurgery.org/surgery/chempeel .htm.
- For an excellent discussion of the appearance of baby's skin at birth, see http://www.childrens.com/HealthLibrary/HealthLibContent.cfm.
- For more information about melanoma, see The American Melanoma Foundation Web site at www.melanomafoundation.org.
- For more information about eczema, see The National Eczema society Web site at www.eczema.org/.
- For more information about psoriasis, see the National Psoriasis Foundation Web site at www.psoriasis.org/.
- For more information about rosacea, see the National Rosacea Society Web site at www.rosacea.org/.
- For information about dermatological disorders as well as a variety of other health problems, see WebMD at www.webmd.com.
- See also http://emedicine.medscape.com/article/1130419-overview for a comprehensive list of Dermatology Internet Sites.

DRUGS

- For information about clinical trials, see www.centerwatch.com. This site also provides a variety of information about clinical research, including a drug directory of FDA-approved medications.
- For safety information about drugs and other products regulated by the U.S. Food and Drug Administration, see www.fda.gov /medwatch.

GENERAL HEALTH

- For information about communicable diseases, see the Web site of the Centers for Disease Control and Prevention (CDC) at www.cdc.gov/.
- For information about ongoing clinical and basic research in dermatology as well as information about dermatological disorders, see www.medscape.com/px/urlinfo.
- For information about prevention and wellness, diseases and conditions, alternative medicine, special health topics, medications, health care providers and facilities, and other information, see The U.S. Department of Health and Human Services at www.hhs.gov. See Healthfinder at www.healthfinder.gov.
- The National Women's Health Information Center at www.4 woman.gov/ provides information about women's health.

- The American Medical Association at www.ama-assn.org/ provides information about a number of health problems and issues.
- For health information, see the Virtual Hospital Web site at www.vh.org/.
- Want to know what those phrases mean on the prescription that your physician wrote for you? For medical and pharmaceutical acronyms and abbreviations, see the Web site of Pharmalexicon at www.pharma-lexicon.com.
- The medical encyclopedia provided by the National Library of Medicine at www.nlm.nih.gov/medlineplus is an excellent resource for additional information about medical conditions, including skin conditions. Pictures are often provided to illustrate skin conditions.
- For information about research in many health areas, see the Web site of the National Institutes of Health at www.nih.gov/.
- For health information and additional databases, see the Web site of the National Library of Medicine at www.nlm.nih.gov/.
- For health information for seniors, see the Web site of NIH Senior Health at www.nihseniorhealth.gov.
- For information on aging, see the Web site of the National Institute on Aging at www.nia.nih.gov/.
- For information about rare diseases, see the Web site of the National Organization for Rare Disorders at www.rarediseases.org.
- For disease overviews and drug information, see the Getting Well Network at www.pdrhealth.com/.
- For medical information about your baby, see the American Academy of Pediatrics Web site at www.aap.org.
- For medical information about many disorders and about fitness, see www.health.harvard.edu.
- For medical information about health issues of minorities, see www.omhrc.gov.

ALTERNATIVE THERAPIES

Listed below are items that are alleged to have certain effects. No attempt is made by this book to verify any of these allegations.

Photoprotection

- Green tea extracts (topical)
- Black tea extracts (topical)
- Ascorbic acid (oral)
- Vitamin E (oral)
- Combination of ascorbic acid, vitamin E, melatonin (topical)

Anti-aging

- Tea produced from leaves of the Eucommia ulmoides Oliver tree (oral) (leaves contain geniposidic acid, reported to enhance skin turnover)
- Spearmint (Mentha spicata): antioxidative effects
- B-Lipohydroxyacid (derivative of salicylic acid): induces epidermal thickening

Treatment for Atopic Dermatitis (Eczema), Psoriasis

- Chinese herbs such as Potentilla chinesis, Tribulus terrestris, Rehmannia glutinosa, Lophatherum gracile, Clematis armandii, Ledebouriella saseloides, Dictamnus dasycarpus, Paeonia lactiflora, Schizonepeta tenuifolia, and Gglabra (herbs boiled to make tea). Combinations of these herbs are reported to have anti-inflammatory, antibacterial, antifungal, antihistamine, and immunosuppressant activities.
- Evening primrose oil (topical): reported helpful to atopic dermatitis
- Borage oil: reported to diminish itching, redness, and oozing of atopic dermatitis
- Oatmeal baths or colloidal oatmeal mixed with liquid (applied topically): reported to relieve itching of atopic dermatitis.
- Ethanol extract from petals of Impatiens balsamina L.: reported helpful in relieving itching of atopic dermatitis
- Furocoumarins (topically or oral) combined with exposure to UVA radiation: helpful to psoriasis (similar to PUVA treatments: psoralin plus UVA)
- Radix (Angelicae dahuricae) (contains the furocoumarins imperatorin, isoimpertorin, and alloimperatorin): treatment of psoriasis
- Camptotheca acuminata decne (used topically with UVA exposure): reported helpful in treatment of psoriasis
- Aloe vera (also reported useful in wound healing): treatment of psoriasis
- Capsaicin (Capiscum frutenscens) (found in cayenne pepper): topical treatment of psoriasis

Treatment for Alopecia Areata

- Lavendar oil
- Aromatherapy with mixture of thyme, rosemary, lavendar, and cedarwood essential oils in jojoba and grape seed carrier oils (rubbed into scalp)

Treatment for Genital Herpes Simplex

- Combination of vitamin E, sodium pyruvate, and membrane-stabilizing fatty acids: reported to be helpful in treating genital herpes simplex in mice and guinea pigs

Treatment for Poison Ivy

- Quaternium-18 bentonite: reported useful in preventing poison ivy reactions

Treatment for Inflammation

- Urtica urens (topical)
- Apis mellifica (topical)
- Belladonna (topical)
- Pulosatilla aqueous gels (topical)
- Arnica montana
- German chamoimile (Matricaria recutita)
- Bittersweet nightshade (S Dulcamara)
- Brewer's yeast (Scerevisia)
- Heartseases (Viola tricolor)
- English plantain (Plantago lanceolata)
- Fenugreek (Trigonella foenum-gaecum)
- Flax (Linum usitatissimum)
- Marshmallow
- Mullein
- Slippery elm

Astringents

- Agrimony (Agrimonia eupatoria)
- Jambolan bark (Syzygium cumini)
- Oak (Quercus rubar)
- Walnut (Juglans regia)
- St John's wort (Hypericum montana)

Treatment for Itching

- Oat straw (A sativa)
- Colloidal oatmeal (oatmeal baths)

Treatment for Acne

- Witch hazel (Hamamelis virginiana) bark extract (topical)
- Fruit acids (citric, gluconic, gluconolactone, glycolic, malic, and tartaric acids) (topical)
- Tea tree oil (oil from the leaves of Melaleuca alternifolia, and Australian tree) (topical)
- Vitex agnus-castus (oral)
- Bittersweet nightshade (Solanum dulcamara) (topical)

- Brewer's yeast (Saccharomyces cervisiae) (oral)
- Topical duckweed (Lemma minor) is used in China to treat acne

Treatment for Warts

- Poldophyllin (from root of American mayapple: Podophyllium) (topical): used to treat venereal warts
- Bittersweet nightshade (S dulcamara) (topical): common warts
- Oat straw (Avena sativa) (topical): common warts
- Calotropis (Calotropis procera): common warts
- Greater celandine (Chelidonium majus): common warts

Wound Healing, Treatment of Burns

- Aloe vera gel (also antibacterial and antifungal, relief of pain and inflammation)
- Marigold (calendula officionalis) (topical): antiseptic, wound healing, diaper dermatitis, ulcers, burns, chapped hands, boils, shingles
- Tannin containing herbs (topical) such as English walnut leaf, goldenrod, Labrador tea, lavender, mullein, oak bark, goldenrod, Labrador tea, lavender, mullein, oak bark, rhatany, Chinese rhubarb, St. John's wort, and yellow dock: astringents (also reported useful in treatment of acne)
- Honey (topical): wound healing, healing of burns, ulcers, infected wounds (antibacterial and antifungal activity)

Laxative

- Aloe vera juice (oral)

Treatment for Fever Blisters (Herpes Simplex)

- Balm (Melissa officinalis) (member of mint family): steam distilled leaves produce oil reportedly helpful in treatment of herpes simplex
- Echinacea (topical)
- Sweet marjoram (topical)
- Peppermint (topical)
- Propolis (topical)

Treatment for Shingles (Herpes Zoster)

- Licorice (Glycyrrhiza glabra, Glycyrrhiza uralensis) gel (topical): shingles and postherpetic neuralgia
- Hibiscus sabdariffa (topical or oral)

Treatment for Infections (Bacterial and Fungal)

- Tea tree oil
- Garlic (topical): fungal infections of feet

Treatment for Scabies, Lice, Other Infestations

Essential oil of anise seeds (Pimpinella anisum): scabies and head lice
Neem (Azadirachta indica) paste, also containing tumeric: scabies, chronic ulcers[2]

NOTES

CHAPTER 3

1. If you have a skin condition such as ichthyosis (dry skin), eczema, or other such disorders, then you may need additional treatment as recommended by your dermatologist.

2. Soaps such as Dove Unscented, Basis, Purpose, or Cetaphil are mild for use on your face as well as on the rest of your body and will sufficiently cleanse your skin.

3. Skin tolerance to products varies with the individual.

4. Moisturizers that are mild and normally function effectively without irritation of skin include Moisturel Lotion, Lubriderm Lotion without lanolin, or Eucerin Lotion.

5. For more information about sun protection, see www.americansun.org.

CHAPTER 4

1. Dermal Gloves.
2. Bristol-Myers Squibb.

CHAPTER 7

1. For illustrations of the different layers of skin and their cells, see the Loyola University Dermatology Medical Education Web site at www.meddean.luc.edu/lumen/MedEd/medicine/dermatology/melton/skinlsn/sknlsn.htm, as well as other Web sites including en.wikipedia.org/wiki/skin.

CHAPTER 8

1. For additional information about treatment of spider veins (sclerotherapy), see http://www.asds-net.org and http://www.plasticsurgery.org/surgery/spidrvns.htm.

2. For more information about facial (chemical) peels, see http://www.asds-net.org and http://www.plasticsurgery.org/surgery/chempeel.htm.

3. Or Jessner's combined with trichloroacetic acid.

4. For additional information about dermabrasion, see http://www.asds-net.org and http://www.plasticsurgery.org/surgery/dermabra.htm.

5. For additional information about laser treatment of vascular lesions or other lesions, see http://www.asds-net.org.

6. For additional information about laser resurfacing, see http://www.asds-net.org and http://www.plasticsurgery.org and http://www.aboardcertifiedplasticsurgeon resource.com/cosmetic/tissue-augmentation/index.html.

7. Pulsed or scanned CO2 lasers and Er:YAG lasers.

8. For additional information on liposuction, see http://www.aboardcertified plasticsurgeonresource.com/liposuction/index.html.

9. For additional information about tissue augmentation, see http://www.aboard certifiedplasticsurgeonresource.com/cosmetic/tissue-augmentation/index.html.

10. McGhan.

11. Ibid.

12. Ibid.

13. LifeCell Corporation.

14. See http://docshop.com/education/dermatology/injectables/fat-transfer/ for more information about micro lipoinjection.

15. DEO-NADGL gel.

16. See http://www.plasticsurgery.org/surgery/hairrepl.htm for further information about hair replacement.

17. Merck & Co.

18. For additional information about blephaloplasty, see http://www .aboardcertifiedplasticsurgeonresource.com/Blepharoplasty/index.html.

19. For more information about electrolysis, see the American Electrology Association Web site at http://electrology.com/.

20. For additional information about laser hair removal, see http://www .aboardcertifiedplasticsurgeonresource.com/laser_hair_removal/index.html.

21. Bristol-Myers Squibb.

22. For more information about retinoids and treatment of wrinkles, see http://www.mayoclinic.com/health/wrinkles/DS00890/DSECTION=treatments-and-drugs.

23. Ortho Dermatological.

24. Botulinum toxin type A (BTX-A, Botox [Allergan]) and botulinum toxin type B (BTX-B, Myobloc [Elan Pharmaceuticals]) are used. BTX-B has faster onset of action than BTX-A, but the duration of BTX-B is shorter. For additional information about botulinum toxin injections, see http://www.mayoclinic.com/health/wrinkles/DS00890/DSECTION=treatments-and-drugs.

CHAPTER 9

1. For more information about sun protection for children, see http://www.medem.com/search/article_display.cfm?path=n:&mstr=/ZZZ9AVFOQ7C.html &soc=AAP&srch_typ=NAV_SERCH.

CHAPTER 10

1. http://www.ncbi.nlm.nih.gov/entrez/query.fcgi.

CHAPTER 11

1. This process of cell death is called "apoptosis."
2. Kagan, V E, Kisin, E R, Kawai, K, Serinkan, B F, Osipov, A N, Serbinova, E A, Wolinsky, I, and Shvedova, A A. Toward mechanism-based antioxidant interventions: lessons from natural antioxidants. *Ann N Y Acad Sci* 2002 Apr;959:188–98.

CHAPTER 12

1. For more information, contact The National Center for Complementary and Alternative Medicine (NCCAM) at the National Institutes of Health (NIH) at its Web site at http://nccam.nih.gov or at the following address:

NCCAM Clearinghouse
P.O. Box 7923
Gaithersburg, Maryland 20898
Toll Free: 1-888-644-6226
International: 301-519-3153
TTY: 1-866-464-3615 **(Toll-Free)**
FAX: 1-866-464-3616 **(Toll-Free)**
Email: info@nccam.nih.gov
2. us.cambridge.org/Books/kiple/introduction1.htm.
3. The Cambridge World History of Food (us.cambridge.org/Books/kiple/introduction1.htm).

CHAPTER 13

1. John E. Bailey, Ph.D., former director of FDA's division of color and cosmetics. From an article by Judith E. Foulke, Staff Writer for FDA consumer, FDA Publication # 95-5013.
2. 2005 IVAX Dermatologicals, Inc.

CHAPTER 14

1. Thomas J. Fitzpatrick, a renowned dermatologist, served as Chairman of Harvard Dermatology for many years.
2. Dr. Richard Glogau, a Harvard Medical School graduate and now a California dermatologist, developed this classification for sun damaged skin.

CHAPTER 15

1. For more information about actinic keratoses, see http://www.skincarephysicians.com/actinickeratosesnet/index.html.
2. For pictures and more information on moles, dysplastic nevi, and melanoma, see http://www.cancer.gov/.

3. For images and more information about melanoma, see http://www.nlm.nih.gov/medlineplus/ency/article/001442.htm.

4. The American Melanoma Foundation (www.melanomafoundation.org/homepage.html) Web site gives excellent information about melanoma.

5. See the National Cancer Institute Web site at http://www.cancer.gov/, for further information on melanoma.

6. For images and additional information about basal cell carcinoma, see http://www.nlm.nih.gov/medlineplus/ency/article/000824.htm.

7. For images and additional information about squamous cell carcinoma, see http://www.nlm.nih.gov/medlineplus/ency/article/000829.htm.

CHAPTER 16

1. For example, isotretinoin (Sotret, Amnesteem).

CHAPTER 17

1. For pictures and information on hair loss and baldness, see http://www.medicinenet.com/hair_loss/article.htm.

2. For pictures and more information on alopecia areata, see http://www.medicinenet.com/alopecia_areata/article.htm.

3. See the National Alopecia Areata Foundation Web site at www.naaf.org for more information about alopecia areata.

4. Rogaine (minoxidil 2%), a topical solution for hair regrowth treatment for men, Rogaine Extra Strength for Men (minoxidil 5%), and Rogaine for Women (minoxidil 2%).

5. Merck & Co.

6. Propecia works by blocking 5-alpha reductase, an enzyme responsible for converting testosterone to dihydro-testosterone (DHT) in males. DHT is an important hormone in male hair loss.

7. For more information about seborrheic dermatitis, see http://www.eczema-assn.org/patiented.html.

8. McNeil Consumer.

9. Westwood Squibb.

10. Ross.

11. Procter & Gamble.

12. Janssen.

13. For more information about hot tub folliculitis, see http://www.nlm.nih.gov/medlineplus/ency/article/001460.htm.

CHAPTER 18

1. For answers to common acne problems, see http://www.medhelp.org/perl6/Dermatology/archive/Acne.html.

2. For cosmetic treatment of acne scars, see http://dermatology.about.com/cs/acnescars/a/acnescars.htm.

3. For images and more information about acne, see http://www.nlm.nih.gov/medlineplus/ency/article/000873.htm.

4. Pharmacia & Upjohn.

5. Emgel (Elan).

6. Dermik.

7. Retin-A Micro 0.1%: Ortho Dermatological.

8. Avita Cream: 0.025% tretinoin cream; Avita Gel: 0.025% tretinoin: Bertek.

9. Tazorac gel 0.05% or 0.1%.

10. Allergan.

11. Galderma.

12. For more information about topical benzoyl peroxide, see http://www
.nlm.nih.gov/medlineplus/druginfo/meds/a601026.html.

13. Stiefel.

14. Oral antibiotics for acne should not be taken during pregnancy.

15. Roche Laboratories.

16. For additional information about isotretinoin, see http://en.wikepedia.org/wiki/
isotretinoin.

17. Retin-A Micro 0.1%: Ortho Dermatological.

18. Allergan.

19. Ibid.

20. Demodex folliculorum

21. Galderma.

22. Ibid.

23. Ibid.

24. Dermik.

25. Azelaic Acid Gel 15%, Intendis.

26. Retin-A.

27. Such as Procter & Gamble, Olay Complete.

28. Moisturel Lotion, Nutraderm Lotion, Purpose moisturizer.

29. Hydroquinone inhibits the conversion of tyrosine to melanin, an important step
in production of skin pigment.

30. Ortho Dermatological.

31. Ibid.

32. Allergan.

33. SalAc

34. Retin-A Micro: Ortho Dermatological.

CHAPTER 19

1. Pfizer Inc., Warner-Lambert Healthcare.

2. Schering-Plough.

3. Ibid.

4. See the Web site of the National Cancer Institute for more information about
papillomaviruses and cancer: www.cancer.gov/cancertopics/factsheet/risk/HPV.

5. Oclassen Pharmaceuticals, Inc.

6. 3M.

7. For pictures and more information about molluscum contagiosum, see http://en
.wikepedia.org/wiki/molluscum_contagiosum.

CHAPTER 20

1. For more information on spider bites, see http://spiders.ucr.edu/.

2. The brown recluse spider, Loxosceles reclusa, is most commonly found in the south central United States. It has a small body with a violin-case pattern on the back and long, delicate legs.

3. The Black widow spider, Latrodectus mactans, is found throughout the United States. Bites in humans occur from the female spider, which has a black shiny body and a red hourglass on its abdomen.

4. For information, see http://www.nlm.nih.gov/medlineplus/ency/article/002860.htm.

5. For more information about lice in the child care setting, see http://kidshealth.org/parent/infections/common/lice.html, http://www.hsph.harvard.edu/headlice.html, and http://www.headlice.org/.

6. Permethrin Cream Rinse: Pfizer Inc., Warner-Lambert Healthcare.

7. Piperonyl Butoxide 4%, Prythrins: Bayer Consumer. In some areas lice are becoming resistant to Nix or Rid. In some cases of such resistance, the dermatologist may need to prescribe topical malathion (Ovide) or topical (1%) or oral ivermectin (Stromectol) to clear the lice.

8. For more information about lice, see http://www.medem.com/medlb/article_detaillb.cfm?article_ID=ZZZ5CPTOBAC&sub_cat=25.

9. Pfizer Inc., Warner-Lambert Healthcare.

10. For pictures and more information about scabies, see http://health.yahoo.com/health/dc/000830/0.html.

11. Alpharma.

12. Bertek.

CHAPTER 21

1. For more information about sun spots, see http://www.skinsite.com/info_lentigine.htm.

2. For pictures and more information about seborrheic keratoses, see http://www.intelihealth.com/IH/ihtIH/WS/9339/10651.html.

3. For more information about skin tags, see http://www.intelihealth.com/IH/ihtIH/WSIHW000/9339/10720.html.

4. Rangel, O, Arias, I, Garcia, E, and Lopez-Padilla, S. Topical tretinoin 0.1% for pregnancy-related abdominal striae: an open-label, multicenter, prospective study. *Adv Ther* 2001 Jul–Aug;18(4):181–6.

5. Nehal, K S, Lichtenstein, D A, Kamino, H, Levine, V J, and Ashinoff, R. Treatment of mature striae with the pulsed dye laser. *J Cutan Laser Ther* 1999 Jan;1(1):41–4.

CHAPTER 22

1. Urushinol.

2. Guttman, C. Systemic CD often an elusive diagnosis. *Dermatology Times*. April 2002, 23(4): 29.

3. Aventis.
4. Schering.
5. Pfizer.
6. Such as Cetaphil soap or unscented Dove soap.
7. Such as Moisturel Lotion or Nutraderm Lotion.
8. Protopic (Fujisawa).
9. Elidel (Novartis Pharmaceuticals).

CHAPTER 23

1. Novartis.
2. Janssen.
3. Medicis.
4. Bertek.
5. Merz.
6. Elan.
7. Schering-Plough.
8. Dermik.
9. Elan.
10. Janssen.
11. Norvartis.
12. Certain drugs may not be taken with itraconazole,. Rarely, congestive heart failure and arrhythymias can occur. Alcoholic beverages should not be consumed while taking antifungal pills, nor should the pills be taken during pregnancy or nursing.
13. For more information about shingles, see http://www.intelihealth.com/IH/ihtIH/WSIHw000/9339/10682.html and http://www.ninds.nih.gov/health_and_medical/disorders/shingles_doc.htm#What_is_Shingles.
14. GlaxoSmithKline.
15. Novartis.
16. GlaxoSmithKline.

CHAPTER 24

1. For images and more information about intertrigo, see http://www.dermnet.org.nz/index.html.
2. Janssen.
3. Person & Covey.
4. Ibid.
5. Allergan.

CHAPTER 25

1. For images and more information about psoriasis, see http://www.intelihealth.com/IH/ihtIH/W/9339/10578.html.
2. For more information about retinoids, see http://www.everydayhealth.com/skin-and-beauty/skin-care-101/retinoids.aspx.

3. Bristol-Myers Squibb Dermatology.

4. Dovonex is a synthetic Vitamin D3 derivative.

5. Neoral gelatin capsules or oral solution: Novartis.

6. CellCept: Roche Laboratories.

7. Soriatane (Acetretin) produced by Roche Laboratories. Soriatane must not be used by females who intend to become pregnant during therapy of any time for at least three years following discontinuation of therapy.

8. Methotrexate slows the abnormally rapid cell turnover seen in psoriasis. Cyclosporine helps suppress the inflammatory reaction in severe, recalcitrant psoriasis. Mycophenolate mofetil inhibits T lymphocyte and B lymphocyte responses to immunological events. Oral retinoids are compounds with vitamin A properties that help cells differentiate properly.

9. Luxiq (betamethasone valerate): Connectics Corporation.

10. Geockerman Treatment.

11. Activated T cells (lymphocytes) play a role in psoriasis.

12. For more information about stasis dermatitis, see http://www.nlm.nih.gov/medlineplus/ency/article/000834.htm.

CHAPTER 26

1. GlaxoSmithKline.

2. Novartis.

3. GlaxoSmithKline.

4. For pictures of herpes simplex including genital herpes infection, see http://www.herpes-coldsores-treatment-pictures.com/.

5. For additional information on canker sores, see http://familydoctor.org/handouts/613.html and http://umm.drkoop.com/conditions/ency/article/001448.htm (picture available).

CHAPTER 27

1. Lee, H J, Ha, S J, Lee, S J, and Kim J, W. Melanocytic nevus with pregnancy-related changes in size accompanied by apoptosis of nevus cells: a case report. *J Am Acad Dermatol* 2000 May;42(5 Pt 2):936–8.

CHAPTER 28

1. For a discussion of baby's skin at birth, see http://www.webmd.com/parenting/baby-skin-care-tips-your-newborn.

2. For information about vascular anomalies, see http://www.birthmarks.us/.

3. For information about mongolian spots, see http://emedicine.medscape.com/article/1068732-overview.

4. For information about atopic dermatitis, see http://www.intelihealth.com/IH/ihtIH/WS/9339/9501.html.

5. For more information about diaper rash, see http://www.mayoclinic.com/health/diaper-rash/ds00069.

6. For image and additional information about impetigo, see http://www.emedicine.com/emerg/topic283.htm#target1 and http://www.medem.com/search/article_display.cfm?path=n:&mstr=/ZZZYDG6G1AC.html&soc=AMA&srch_typ=NAV_SERCH.

CHAPTER 31

1. Methotrexate acts by slowing down "cell turnover" in skin. "Cell turnover" is the skin's way of rejuvenating itself by producing new cells to replace the old. In normal skin this is a valuable function; in psoriasis this occurs too rapidly, resulting in thick skin plaques of psoriasis.

2. Amevive (human LFA3-IgG fusion protein).

3. Remicade (Centocor).

4. Embrel (Wyeth-Ayerst Laboratories).

5. Arava (Aventis).

6. Leflunomide is a pyrimidine synthesis inhibitor that blocks T cell clonal expansion.

7. Liver damage has occurred in some patients taking leflunomide. Etanercept has been associated with rare cases of pancytopenia including aplastic anemia. There have also been rare reports of demyelinating disorders including multiple sclerosis, myelitis, and optic neuritis, with some patients taking etanercept. Etanercept and infliximab have been associated with development of infections. There have been reports of activation of tuberculosis in some patients receiving infliximab. Treatments with these new medications are being carefully monitored.

8. Fujisawa.

9. Novartis.

10. The 0.1% concentration of tacrolimus is FDA approved for use in adults. The lower 0.03% concentration is approved for use in both children (ages two and above) and adults for short-term and intermittent long-term treatment.

11. There is risk of lymphoma with long-term use of Elidel.

12. Aldara (3M corporation) is FDA approved for treatment of genital warts, actinic keratoses (precancers of skin), and superficial basal cell skin cancers.

13. Allergan.

14. VASER LipoSelection (ISIS).

15. Ultrashape.

16. SlipLipo (Palomar).

17. Guttman, C. Dermal fillers on horizon, offer new benefits. *Dermatology Times.* April 2002: 23(4):55.

18. Other hormonal acne treatments include anti-androgens such as spironolactone or flutamide. Spironolactone and flutamide block the effects of testosterone on the sebaceous glands and the hair follicle. There is less oil production and facial hair growth, resulting in improvement of acne and lessening of excessive hair growth.

19. Phizer. Approved July 2001.

20. Ortho Pharmaceutical Corporation.

21. Acticoat (Westaim Biomedical).

22. ProCyte Corp.

23. Ortho-McNeil.

24. Bryant, R. Skin substitutes surge ahead. *Dermatology Times*. April 2002: (23)4:41.

25. From the outer root sheath of the hair

26. N-2-butylcyanoacrylate (GluStitch).

27. AstraZeneca. For more information about EMLA, see www.emla-us.com.

28. Such as methemoglobinemia, where an abnormal hemoglobin state exists such that the hemoglobin does not transport oxygen.

29. Emla should not be used in children with methemoglobinemia or in infants under the age of 12 months who are receiving treatment with methemoglobin-inducing agents.

30. The Gebauer Company.

31. Iomed.

32. Epidermal barrier.

33. Bioject (www.bioject.com), Injex (www.equidyne.com), Antares (www .antarespharma.com) are only a few of many companies involved in this endeavor.

34. Sator, P G, Schmidt, J B, Sator, M O, Huber, J C, and Honigsmann, H. The influence of hormone replacement therapy on skin ageing: a pilot study. *Maturitas* 2001 Jul 25;39(1):43–55.

35. 9th International Congress on Anti-Aging & Biomedical Technologies, Dec. 14–16,2001.

36. Sauerbronn, A V, Fonseca, A M, Bagnoli, V R, Saldiva, P H, and Pinotti J A. The effects of systemic hormonal replacement therapy on the skin of postmenopausal women. *Int J Gynaecol Obstet* 2000 Jan;68(1):35–41.

37. Brincat, M P. Hormone replacement therapy and the skin. *Maturitas* 2000 May 29;35(2):107–17.

38. EndoVenous Laser Treatment.

39. Eg. containing antioxidant vitamin C, Vitamin E, or coenzyme Q10. Antioxidants work to protect skin from breakdown of collagen, caused by aging and by sunlight.

40. Copper-containing cosmetics are reported to improve not only skin appearance but also skin elasticity, thickness, and firmness.

41. Such as Dove for Sensitive Skin, Cetaphil, Basis.

42. Such as Moisturel Lotion, Eucerin Lotion, Lubriderm Lotion.

43. Such as Anthelios, Solbar.

44. From the fruit of the Coffea Arabica plant.

CHAPTER 32

1. Imiquimod is also FDA approved for treatment of skin precancers and genital warts.

CHAPTER 33

1. Ahmad, W, Faiyaz, U L, Haque, M, et al. Alopecia universalis associated with a mutation in the human hairless gene. *Science*. 1998; 279:720–724.

2. Some viruses contain RNA (ribonucleic acid) instead of DNA.

3. SNP's (small nucleoproteins).

4. Many are concerned that such knowledge may affect their ability to obtain health insurance or jobs. Lawmakers are now at work to prevent discrimination on the basis of genetic testing.

CHAPTER 34

1. Under President George Bush.

2. Shinya Yamanaka, Tokyo University.

3. James A. Thompson, University of Wisconsin-Madison.

4. *Oct ¾, Sox2, c-Myc, Klf4*

5. Liang, L, and Bickenbach, J R. Somatic epidermal stem cells can produce multiple cell lineages during development. *Stem Cells* 2002;20(1):21–31.

6. Science, August 29, 2008.

7. Nature, August 27, 2008.

8. *C-Myc.*

9. Retrovirus.

10. Adenovirus.

CHAPTER 35

1. Khademhosseini, A, Vacanti, J P, and Langer, R. "Progress in Tissue Engineering." *Scientific American.* May 2009.

2. Ibid.

3. Ali Khademhosseini, Joseph P. Vacanti, Robert Langer.

CHAPTER 36

1. Mallouk, T E, and Sen, A. Powering Nanorobots. *Scientific American*, May 2009.

2. James Tour, Rice University.

3. Thomas E Mallouk, Ayusman Sen, Pennsylvania State University *Scientific American*, May 2009.

4. Rustem Ismagilov, George Whitesides.

APPENDIX

1. It is important that blood cell count and liver function tests are monitored if such herbal treatment is utilized.

2. Can be poisonous to children.

REFERENCES

Alster, T S, and Lupton, J R. Update on Dermatologic Laser Surgery: New Trends for 2002. *Cosmetic Dermatology* 2002 Feb;15(2):33–36.

American Academy of Dermatology Annual Meeting: San Francisco 2009.

American Academy of Dermatology: www.aad.org.

American Academy of Facial Plastic and Reconstructive Surgery: www.aafprs.org.

American Society for Dermatologic Surgery: www.asds-net.org/.

Arndt, K A, LeBoit, P E, Robinson, J K, and Wintroub B U, editors. *Cutaneous Medicine and Surgery*, First Edition. Philadelphia:W.B. Saunders; 1996.

Bedi, M K, and Shenefelt, P D. Herbal Therapy in Dermatology. *Arch Dermatol* 2002 Feb; 138:232–242.

Bowers, J. Getting personal: The promise of genomic medicine. *Dermatology World*; Jan. 2009.

CenterWatch/Clinical Trials Listing.

CenterWatch/Clinical Trials Listing Service: www.centerwatch.com/patient/drugs.

Draelos, Z. Cosmeceuticals in the Rosacea Patient. *Cosmetic Dermatology*. 2002 Feb;15; (2):48.

Draelos, Z D. Cosmetic Conundrums. *Dermatology Times* 2002 Mar; 23(3):58.

Draelos, Z D. Optimal Skin Care for Aesthetic Patients: Topical Products to Restore and Maintain Healthy Skin. *Cosmetic Dermatology*; March 2009: 22(3).

Edwards, M. Beneath the Surface of Scars and Wound Healing. Healthy Skin & Hair. 2001 Winter; Supp. To *Cosmetic Dermatology*; p11.

Fitzpatrick, T B, Eisen, A Z, Wolff, K, Freedberg, I M, and Austen, K F, editors. *Dermatology in General Medicine*, Fourth Edition. New York: McGraw-Hill;1993.

Goldman, M. Cellulite: A Review of Current Treatments. *Cosmetic Dermatology*. 2002 Feb; 15(2):17.

Levin, C, and Maibach, H. 2002. Exploration of "Alternative" and "Natural" Drugs in Dermatology. *Arch Dermatol* 2002 Feb;138:207–211.

Mallouk, T E, and Sen, A. Powering Nanorobots. *Scientific American* May 2009.

Matarasso, S L. Skin Resurfacing. Csr 106, New Orleans American Academy of Dermatology 60th Annual Meeting, Feb 22–27, 2002.

Nasir, A. Review of Nanoparticles, Part I. *Cosmetic Dermatology* March 2009, 22(3).

The National Center for Complementary and Alternative Medicine (NCCAM) at the National Institutes of Health: http://nccam.nih.gov.

Pollard, K S. What Makes Us Human? *Scientific American* May 2009.

Pribitkin, E D, and Boger, G. Herbal therapy: what every facial plastic surgeon must know. *Arch Facial Plast Surg* 2001 Apr–Jun; 3(2):127–32.

Schwanke, J. ALA/PDT therapy branches toward benign skin tumors. *Dermatology Times* 2000 Mar;23(3):30.

Shoemaker, B. Noninvasive fat removal looms on cosmetic horizon. *Dermatology Times* 2000 Mar; 23(3): 66.

Siegel, D M. Opening the Doors of Perception: Complementary Approaches to Dermatologic Diseases. *Arch Dermatol* 2002 Feb;138:251–253.

INDEX

Accutane, 118
Acid: alpha-hydroxy, 63; azelaic, 119,
    123–24; hyaluronic, 47
acne, 42, 44–45, 66, 117–25, 165, 185–
    86; adult, 4; cysts, 121;
    inflammatory, 119–20;
    isotretinoin treatment, 118;
    medications, 14; scars, 42;
    treatment, laser, 90
acne neonatorum, 165
actinic keratoses, 41, 100, 105, 185
action plan for healthy skin, 88
acyclovir, 148, 150, 161
Addison's disease, 155
advertising hype, 67–68, 202, 212
aesthetician, 41
agent, photosensitizing, 101
aging, 112, 190, 201; skin changes, 35
ALA (5-aminolevulinic acid), 185
albinism, 199
allergic reactions, 40, 47, 141–42
allergies, 24, 153
AlloDerm, 47
Aloe vera, 67–68, 156
alopecia areata, 112, 115
alpha-hydroxy acid products, 63
alternative medicines, 71
alternative therapies, 67–71
aluminum chloride, 152
amazing skin, 27–33
amazing transformations, 40
angiogenesis, 175
angular chelitis (cracks in corners of
    mouth), 162

Anthelios, 12
antibiotics, 154, 158, 185
anticancer possibilities, 196
antihistamines, 84, 140, 142, 153
antioxidants, 63–65, 141, 190, 210
antiperspirant, 152
appearance: transformations, 39–40;
    youthful, 32, 37, 39, 48–49,
    86, 95
areas: diaper, 167; hair-bearing, 112,
    145; irritated, 140, 149, 167;
    white, 154
aromatherapy, 65–66, 94, 96
artificial tanning products, 176
astringents, 42
at-home laser hair removal devices, 215
atopic dermatitis, 143, 166, 181, 191
attack cells, 196–97
avobenzone, 12

baby's skin, 54
balanced diet, 20, 71, 84, 88–96
balding scalps, 182
bandages, 187
barrier, 11; physical, 27; protection, 35
basal cell carcinoma, 104–5
basement membrane, 27, 29, 31, 37, 210
basics: for beautiful skin, 9; of skin care,
    83
benadryl, 140, 153
benzoyl peroxide products, 121
bimatoprost ophthalmic solution, 183
bioengineered human collagen products,
    184

biologics, 166, 176–77, 180
biopsy, 104–5, 139
birthmarks, 165
bites, 131–33, 168; mosquito, 159, 168;
    spider, 131–32
bleaching creams, 61, 119, 124
blephlaroplasty, 49
blood cells, white, 29
blood vessels, little, 122–23
body lice, 132
boils, 154
borders, vermillion, 154–55
Botox, 39, 51, 74, 86, 152, 219
brown recluse spider, 131
building up from the basics, 15
burn, razor, 114

calcium alginate, 187
cancer cells, 196–97, 211
C. elegans, learning from the worm, 193
cell differentiation, 217
cells: cancerous, 181, 196, 210;
    dendritic, 195; destroy
    precancerous, 101; differentiated,
    203; embryonic, 205; fly, 195
cell signals, 32, 207, 210
cell turnover, 74
cellulite, 51, 57; treatment, 51
checkups, regular, 25, 86, 96, 128
chemical peels, 39, 95, 120, 135
ciclopirox, 145–46
claims, exaggerated, 73
Clarisonic Skin Care Brush, 73
cleansers, effective skin, 190
cleansing, 60, 87
collaborations, 171, 173, 175, 191
collagen, 32, 35, 37, 44, 47, 210; cow,
    47; human, 47, 184; human
    bioengineered, 47
companies, pharmaceutical, 60–61, 177,
    182, 191
complexion, 35, 83, 92, 189
contraceptives, 119, 186
cosmeceuticals, 190–91, 212
cosmetic procedures, 39
cosmetics, 189

cracks, 17–18, 20, 109, 162
cradle cap, 113, 167
creams: antifungal, 145, 147; antiscabies,
    133; antiwrinkle, 36, 73–74;
    anti-yeast, 114, 147; imiquimod,
    128, 197; steroid, 112, 137, 140,
    158; wrinkle-cure, 51
crust: thick, 113; yellow, 168
cuticles, 19
cycle, itch-scratch, 159
cysts, 84, 118, 154
cytokines, 32

damage, 13
damaged cells, replacing, 204–5
dandruff, 113, 146
danger signs of skin cancer, 101
dark patches, 42, 61, 119, 123–24,
    163
dark spots, 41, 63, 95, 110, 119, 135
dead skin, clearing, 41
defective gene products, 201
defensins, 186
dermabrasion, 39, 42–43, 188
dermatitis: contact, 139, 141; seborrheic,
    113–14, 146, 167
dermis, 27, 31–32, 37, 103, 175, 210
destroy fat cells, 183–84
development of new blood vessels,
    175
DHT, 112
diapers, changing, 17
diet, well-balanced, 24, 51, 64–65
discoveries: new, 58, 171–72, 181, 190,
    193, 212; scientific, 58, 193,
    202, 212
disorders: autoimmune, 196; inherited,
    201
DNA, 99, 194, 199–200, 202; damaged,
    65, 99–100; human, 194; worm's,
    194
dry lips, 109
dry skin, 109–10, 153, 159
Dry Touch (Ultra Sheer), 13
ducts, sebaceous, 117
dysplastic moles, 101–2

eczema, 24, 115, 142–43, 166–67, 181
effective sun protection, 13
Efudex, 100
elasticity, 31–32, 35, 74, 189–90
elastin, 31–32, 35–36, 44, 210
elbows, 17–21, 127, 157, 166
electrolysis, 50
Elidel, 166–67, 181
embryos, 203–4; human, 204
EMLA, 188
epidermis, 27–32, 35, 37, 42–45
era, incredible, 201
Etanercept, 180
eternal youthfulness, 25, 58
examination, full-skin, 101
excision, 105, 164
exercise program, 24, 84
eyebrows, 92, 115
eyelashes, 15, 183
eyelids, 51, 86, 140, 183
eye makeup, 86, 95–96

facial: blemishes, 117–25; peels, 41–42,
    91, 93, 95, deep, 41, medium
    depth, 41, superficial, 41; redness,
    92–93, 123, 155; resurfacing, 39,
    50, 95–96; sagging, 74; skin lift,
    49; skin resurfacing, 45
facials, 42, 63, 65–66, 88
facial skin: smooth, 95; tighten, 44
Famvir, 148, 150, 161
fat, excess, 183
fat cells, 51, 183
FDA (Federal Drug Administration)
    approval, 58, 68–69, 73, 180, 188
feet, 17–18, 148; sweating, 51
fever blisters, 21, 24, 161
fibers, elastic, 37
fibroblasts, 31–32, 35–36, 45, 175, 209
fillers, 184, 219
fine wrinkles, 47, 50, 64, 73, 209
fingernails, 19, 145–46
fingertips, 18
Fitzpatrick skin types, 79
flaking scalps, 112, 147
folliculitis, 114

foot, athlete's, 19, 146–47
foundation makeup, 10, 85–87, 90–93,
    95–96
fragrance, 11
Fraxel, 45, 86, 88, 95–96
free radicals, 64–65
fresh skin appearance, 23
fruit fly, learning from, 194

genes: cancer-causing, 211; defective,
    200–201; functions, 194; therapy,
    172
genetic code, 197
goals, 87
golden rule of skin care, 15

hair: care of, 17; eyebrow, 115; gray, 50,
    215; problems with, 111; removal,
    215; substitute, 187; thinning, 48,
    111, 133, 182
hair cycle, 191, 215
hair follicles, 36, 112–15, 171–72,
    182
hair growth: anagen phase, 113, 182–83;
    catagen phase, 182; excessive, 115;
    facial, 50; slowing with Vaniqa,
    50; telogen phase, 113, 182
hair loss, 111–13, 115, 118, 182, 215
hair removal, 50; with electrolysis, 50;
    with laser, 50
hair transplantation, 48, 112
hands, care of, 17–18
health, good, 23
healthy body, 23, 65, 79, 84
healthy skin program, 79–96
heat, prickly (miliaria rubra), 155
helioplex, 12
hemangiomas, 44, 165; laser treatment,
    44; strawberry, 165
herbal product, 71
herpes gestationis, 163
herpes simplex, 149, 162
herpes zoster, 148
hidradenitis suppurativa, 153–54
hirsutism, 114–15
hives, 141–42

hormones, 35, 112–13, 117–18, 186, 189
hot areas of scientific research, 175–77
human DNA code, 197
Hydraphase UV, 30, 12
hydroquinone, 119, 124, 190
hyperpigmentation, post-inflammatory, 119
hypertrophic, 137

imiquimod, 100, 181
immune cells, 29–30, 128, 177, 179–81, 186, 194
immune system, 27, 106, 177, 181, 185, 194–96; acquired, 195–96
immunomodulators, 176–77, 180–81
impetigo, 168
implants, 47–48, 208
infection: bacterial, 139, 194; fungal, 19–20, 145–48
infestation, 153
inflammation, 100, 120, 143, 158, 185–86, 196
infliximab, 180
ingredients, natural, 67–68, 156
injectable: human collagen products, 184; poly-L-lactic acid product, 184
intense pulsed light (IPL) treatment, 45, 50, 86, 95
interleukins, 181
intertrigo, 151
intrinsic aging, 36–37, 95
iontophoresis, 152, 188
irritation of hands and feet, 17
isotretinoin, 45, 83, 118–19, 154
itching, 132–33, 141, 143, 153, 159

jock itch, 147
Juvaderm, 184

keratinocytes, 28–30, 37
ketoconazole, 113–14, 145, 151

Lamisil, 145–46
Langerhans cells, 29–30, 37
large pores, 91, 124–25

laser: body sculpting, 184; hair removal, 50, 215; resurfacing, 39, 44–45
Latisse, 183
layer, basal, 28–31, 37
layers, upper skin, 155
leflunomide, 180
lentigines, 85
lentigo maligna, 135
lesions, psoriatic, 179
lice, 131–32, 153
lichen simplex chronicus, 158–59
lidocaine, 47, 102, 104, 188
light: blue, 101, 120; infrared, 211; power of, 101, 186; ultraviolet, 121, 157–58, 179
light spots, 110, 150
lip definition, 184
liposuction, 39, 46–47, 51, 183–84; techniques, 184
lips, 154; dark lines around, 154
lipstick, 21, 46–47, 91–92, 109, 154
liquid nitrogen, 100, 127, 129, 135–36, 184
losing hair, 111
loss of skin color, 154
lymphocytes, 179, 181

macrophages, 65
makeup, 13, 41, 87–88, 90, 93, 154
massage, 24, 42, 51, 66, 94
medical: information, 60; offices, 213, 215; problems, 25, 42, 59, 70, 112, 202; tourism, 213–14
medicines, 70–71, 84, 139, 141–42, 158, 210
melanocytes, 30, 35, 176–77
melanoma, 20, 101–3, 135, 164, 211, 217; cells, 211; and pregnancy, 164; reactivation of, 164
melasma, 123–24, 163
mexoryl, 12
microdermabrasion, 43, 73, 88, 95–96, 120, 219
Microsporum canis, 145
minoxidil, 112, 182

mites, 131, 133
moisturizers, 11, 18–19, 53, 73, 80
moles, 101–3, 106, 163; abnormal, 101; evolving, 101–2; removal, 102
molluscum contagiosum, 128
MRSA (Methicillin resistant staphlococcus aureus), 149
myths, 63–66

nail changes, 20
nails, 18, 146; thick, 146
nanometers, 209
nanoparticles, 209–12
nanotechnology, 211
natural products, 42, 58, 68
neck, sagging, 86
nerve cells, 31, 203, 205; motor, 204–5
new blood vessels, 175
newborn skin, 53
new breakthroughs, 179, 190–91
new genomic era, 201; impact on skin, 202
new products, innovative, 60, 197
new wound-healing products, 187
nipples, 114–15
nits, 132

oil, mineral, 18–20, 109, 166–67
over-the-counter products, 58, 121, 162
oxiconazole nitrate, 145–46
oxidative stress, 65

PABA, 14
parsol, 12
patch, herald, 143
patch test, 141
PDT, 101, 185
pencil, eyebrow, 115
perfume, 11, 94
perfumed soaps, 11, 91, 93–94, 152
permethrin, 133
peroxide: benzoyl, 118, 121, 124; hydrogen, 102, 124, 137, 210–11
petroleum jelly, 109–10
photoaging, 12, 37, 85; protection from, 14

photopneumatic therapy, 120
photoprotection, 74; the future, 176
pigment cells, 35, 110
pityriasis rosea, 143
plantar warts, 127, 185
PML (progressive multifocal leukoencephalopathy), 180
poison ivy, 139
poison ivy plant, 140
poison sumac, 141
pores, clogged, 86, 119
port wine stains, 44, 165; laser treatment, 44
precancers, 41, 85–86, 90, 95–96, 100–101
pregnancy, 124, 157, 163
preparations, skin bleaching, 124
preventing sun damage, 14, 31, 54, 85–86, 95, 101
products: alpha-hydroxy, 123; anti-aging, 59; bleaching, 124; breakthrough, 74–75, 202; non-perfumed, 159; redness-relief, 156; sulfur-based, 121; tretinoin, 64, 124
Propecia, 49, 112, 182
protection, excellent, 12
protective clothing, 14, 54, 100
Protopic, 166–67, 181
protoporphyrins, 186
psoralin, 158
psoriasis, 21, 157–58, 163, 179–81; treating, 157–58, 180, 191
pubic region, 132
pulsed light, intense, 45, 50, 86, 95, 219
pumice stone, 127–28
PUPPP, 163
PUVA, 158

Raptiva, 180
rash: diaper, 167; drug, 141; itchy, 139–40, 163, 166; red, 67, 147
reactions: allergic contact, 140; id, 148–49; systemic, 132

recovery time, 41, 43, 45–46, 184
rectal itch, 151
redness, relieve, 155–56
reformulating old products, 171
regular skin check-ups, 135, 164
relax wrinkles, 39, 51
removing skin cancers, 99
Renova, 50, 64, 73, 124
research, hot areas, 191
research bench to product, 172
Restylane, 43, 47, 184
rhinophyma, 122
ringworm, 143, 145
Rogaine, 112
rosacea, 117–18
roseola, 168
rubber gloves, 17

salicylic acid, 41, 113–14, 121, 124,
    127; plasters, 127, 137; products,
    121; wash, 80
saline, hypertonic, 40
saliva, 20, 162
Sarna Lotion, 143, 155, 159, 168
scabies, 132–33, 153
scalp: baby's, 113, 167; conditions, 20,
    112; hairs, 115; psoriasis, 157;
    reduction, 48, 112
scars, 45, 47, 105, 121, 125, 136–37;
    keloid, 137
scientists: academic, 60, 175, 182;
    industry, 175; university, 171
sclerotherapy, 40, 189
scratching, 20
Sculptra, 88, 95–96, 184
sebaceous glands, 36, 66, 120
seborrheic keratoses, 86, 135–36, 185
sebum, 117
self-renewing stem cells, 203
sensational skin, 23–25
sensitive skin, 89–90, 162
sensitivity, 140
sensitivity to a product, 10, 18, 141–42
septa, fibrous, 51
shampoo, gentle, 53
shingles, 147–48

shooting pains, 147–48
side effects of laser treatment, 44
signs, danger in moles, 101–2
size, pore, 124–25
skin: alligator, 21; baby, 53; basic care,
    64; the body's protector, 27;
    brown, 79; changes in pregnancy,
    163; common problems in
    children, 166; dangers of sun
    exposure, 99; dark, 79, 104; exam,
    regular, 99; exfoliating, 120;
    firming, 95–96; firmness, 31–32,
    35, 74, 189; glowing, 25; habits,
    bad, 87; healthy, 24, 64, 87, 190;
    healthy body-healthy skin, 84;
    irritated, 109, 151, 158, 162; irri-
    tation, 11, 18, 151; lax, 51;
    lighten, 124; mottled, 110; new,
    44, 204; oily, 80, 124; olive, 79,
    91; photoaged, 44; a physical
    barrier, 27; plan, daily, 88; psori-
    atic, 180; radiant, 25; rash, 168;
    resurface, 43; sagging, 24, 47, 95;
    scaling, 21; self-examination, 107;
    sensational, 26; sensitivity, 14,
    140; sensitivity to products in
    sunscreens, 14; as a sensory organ,
    27; smooth, 39, 73; soothe, 58,
    175; sun-damaged, 43, 63;
    sun-exposed, 185; tanning dam-
    ages, 176; thick, 19, 21; turnover,
    39, efficient, 37; upper layer of,
    42–43, 74; white, 79, 94; wrin-
    kling, 37, 175; young, 36
skin aging, 35–37, 86, 175; extrinsic, 36;
    intrinsic, 36; premature with sun
    exposure, 37; reversible causes, 36;
    signs of, 36, 41
skin barrier, 11; harm, 17
skin biopsy, 104
skin cancer, important information,
    99
skin cancers:
basal cell, 104, 197; deadly, 99;
    developing, 85, 87, 110; increased
    risk of, 54, 158

Skin Care Brush, 73
skin cells: communication, 32;
    fibroblasts, 31; keratinocytes, 29;
    Langerhans cells, 29; melanocytes,
    30; nerve cells, 31
skin layers, 28, 31, 217; basal layer, 28;
    dermis, 27; epidermis, 28
skin lifts, 49
skin replacement, permanent, 208
skin substitutes, 187
skin tags, 136
skin talk signals, 210
skin type, 79, 88–89, 91, 94
soap, antibacterial, 10, 18, 166
Solaraze, 100
solar lentigines, 135
sores: canker, 161–62; cold, 42, 45, 148–
    49, 161–62
Soriatane, 157
Sotradecol, 40
spas, 63, 65–66, 213, 215
SPF (sun protective factor), 12–13, 54,
    85, 93–95, 100
spiders, 131
spots: bald, 35, 48, 182; mongolian, 166
squamous cell carcinoma, 104–5
stasis dermatitis, venous, 158
stem cell research, 205
stem cells: adult, 203–4; embryonic,
    203–5, 207; human, 204; induced
    pluripotent, 204; precursor, 204;
    reprogram, 204; somatic, 203
stings, bee, 131
stress-buster break, 24–25
stretch marks, 74, 137
subcutaneous fat, layer of, 27
substances, natural, 57, 67
sunblocks, 13–14
sunburn, 14, 199, 217
sunglasses, 14, 37, 79, 89–90, 94–95
sun protection, 12, 54
sunscreen, 11–14, 61, 81, 91, 94, 100
sunscreens are not all alike, 13

sunscreens with micronized particles, 13
sun sensitivity with medications, 14

sun spots, 99, 135
sweating, 51; hands, 51
swelling, leg, 158

tanning, 14, 36–37
tanning beds, skin risks, 37
tattoo removal, 188–89
technology: new, 189–90, 194, 215;
    taking home, 215
telangectasia, 86, 104, 122–23, 163,
    189
telogen effluvium, 111
therapies, new, 176–77, 193, 201,
    205
tinea versicolor, 150
tissue augmentation, 39, 46–47
tissue-engineered products, developing,
    208
tissue transplantation, 205
T-lymphocytes, 181, 186
toenails, 18–19, 145–46
toes, 18–19, 146–47, 151
transplantation, hair, 48, 177, 203,
    207–8
tretinoin, 50, 64, 129, 137
truth about skin, 57, 202
truth or illusion, distinguishing, 59
tubs, hot, 114

underarms, 51
UVA (ultraviolet A), 12, 68, 190
UVB (ultraviolet B), 12, 14, 158, 190
UV Expert 20, 12
UV Light Boxes, 157–58

Valtrex, 148, 150, 161
Vaniqa, 50
Vaseline, 18, 21, 102, 137
Vectical, 157, 180
veins, leg, injections, 39–40, 189. See also
    sclerotherapy
virus, herpes, 21, 148, 162–63
vitamin D, 217
vitamin preparations, 63–64
vitiligo, 154
Vytone Cream, 151–52

warts, 105, 127–28, 136, 181, 184–85;
     genital, 128
wash, 10, 20, 87, 121, 132; benzoyl
     peroxide, 114, 121
washing your face, 10
white patches of skin, 154
wound healing, 33, 64, 74, 175, 186

wrinkles: erasing, 95–96; reduction, 45,
     50

Xeroderma pigmentosa, 201

Zovirax, 148, 150, 161

About the Author

Rebecca B. Campen, M.D., obtained an M.D. at the Medical College of Georgia in 1987, a J.D. at the University of Georgia School of Law in 1983, and completed a residency in dermatology at the Medical College of Georgia in 1991. She is a Fellow of the American Academy of Dermatology (AAD), served as AAD Liaison to the Federal Trade Commission, and served on the AAD Regulatory Committee.

Dr. Campen is involved in teaching and training of medical students and residents as Assistant Professor of Dermatology at Harvard Medical School. She has served as Chief of Staff of the Harvard Department of Dermatology, Deputy Director of the Massachusetts General Hospital/Harvard Cutaneous Biology Research Center, and member of the Executive Committee of Harvard Dermatology. She has served on the MGH Quality Assurance Committee, the MGH Compliance Committee, the MGH Patient Care Assessment Committee, and the MGH Institutional Review Board. She has been involved in dermatological care at the Massachusetts General Hospital in Boston since 1991, and currently divides her time between her clinical activities in Boston and her private office, Campen Dermatology, in Savannah, Georgia.

Dr. Campen is the author of two previous books, *Going into Medical Practice* and *Blueprints in Dermatology*.